Counselling in a
General Practice Setting

Gateways to Counselling

Consultant editor:
Windy Dryden, Professor of Counselling at Goldsmiths College,
University of London

Series editor:
Maria Stasiak

Project manager:
Carron Staplehurst

The *Gateways to Counselling* series comprises books on various aspects of counselling theory and practice. Written with the assistance of the Central School of Counselling and Therapy, one of the largest counselling training organisations in the UK, the books address the needs of both students and tutors and are relevant for a range of training courses, regardless of specific orientation.

Other books in the series include:

STARVING TO LIVE
The paradox of anorexia nervosa
Alessandra Lemma-Wright

AN INTRODUCTION TO CO-DEPENDENCY FOR
COUNSELLORS
Gill Reeve

COUNSELLING SKILLS FOR PROFESSIONAL HELPERS
John Pratt

ON LISTENING AND LEARNING
Student counselling in further and higher education
Colin Lago and Geraldine Shipton

TRANSCULTURAL COUNSELLING
Zack Eleftheriadou

COUNSELLING IN A GENERAL PRACTICE SETTING

James Breese

Central Book Publishing Ltd
London

First published 1994
by Central Book Publishing Ltd
Centre House, 56B Hale Lane
London, NW7 3PR

© 1994 James Breese

Phototypeset in 10 on 12 point Century Roman and Optima by
Intype, London
Printed in Great Britain by
Tudor Printing, Park Rd, Barnet

Cover illustration by Helen S. Roper

British Library Cataloguing in Publication Data

Breese, James
Counselling in a General Practice
Setting. – (Gateways to Counselling
Series)
I. Title II. Series
362.104256

ISBN 1–898458–10–3

Contents

Introduction

I was asked to write this book because for the past nine years I have organised, counselled in and done much of the individual supervision of colleagues in a counselling agency located in a GPs' surgery. The growth and work of this agency is fully described in Chapter 5, but it is my experience of work in this setting as well as my previous work as a RELATE counsellor for over twenty years and my experience of teaching it at Diploma and Certificate levels that qualifies me to write on this subject.

Why write a book specifically about counselling in the setting of a GPs' surgery? One answer is that it has become very evident in the last few years that many GPs welcome the idea of having a counsellor attached to their surgery. For many patients, seeing a counsellor in a setting which is familiar is easier than having to contact a separate agency and go to an unfamiliar location. And in the words of one of the three GPs who have made invaluable contributions to this book, referring a patient to a counsellor one knows is more satisfactory than referring them to a stranger.

Counsellors need to be trained and there are many extensive training courses available. What is difficult to know for certain is how much initial training a counsellor needs before seeing clients. What is as crucial as any initial training is the on-going training that all counsellors should be experiencing through regular groups for case discussion and through individual supervision. The experience of having been counselled is also very desirable, some would say essential.

It is difficult at this stage of the development of surgery counselling to know whether there are specific topics peculiar to counselling in surgeries which ought to be addressed on training courses. The evidence so far, from a study mentioned in Chapter 1, is that training institutions have not seriously addressed this matter.

The case for having a counsellor as part of the surgery team is established in Chapter 1 where I am very indebted to the contributions from two GPs, Dr Roger Burford and Dr Iain Duncan. Chapter 2 considers the type of problems clients bring, how to help those recommended for counselling but who are reluctant to come, and the liaison between the counsellor and the GPs and other members of the surgery team. Chapter 3 deals with practicalities, including whether being on medication hinders the counselling process, and in Chapter 4 consideration is given to the kinds of research that have so far been done. Chapter 5 is an account of the work of the charity Off the Record Norfolk and Norwich Counselling Agency which over the past eight years has grown from 3 counsellors giving between them 265 appointments a year, to 22 counsellors giving over 2,500 appointments.

As well as the increase in the work of this agency, where most of the work is voluntary, the years 1991 and 1992 saw a considerable increase in counselling in GPs' surgeries when payment to the counsellors became available through funding for Health Promotion Clinics. Counselling was recommended more and more by GPs and waiting lists in other surgeries grew and grew. Maybe counselling became a victim of its own success. A change in NHS policy whereby the Health Promotion Clinic Scheme was abandoned, except for clinics for certain specific ailments, has led to a reduction in the amount of counselling in other surgeries in the area where I work, despite an increase in demand from patients. There is thus currently a crisis for patients and for counsellors and considerable strain on the resources of voluntary agencies.

In addition to the GPs already mentioned above, I am indebted to Dr Sue Vaughan for her contribution in Chapter 5 and to the following counselling colleagues who work either in the surgery setting described in Chapter 5 or in other surgeries in Norfolk and elsewhere: Brian Bassingthwaighte, Sue Bayliss, Jackie Bullimore, Nina Cowan, Sheila Cree, Simon Frey, Jennifer Harrison, Richard House, Jacqui Hughes, Yvonne Poles, Jo Rivett, Garth Stacey, Ros Staveley and Peter

Varney. Where appropriate, their names have been altered in the text as have the names of any clients to whose cases I have referred. Without the contact with these last and without the support of the counselling colleagues mentioned by name and many others over the years, this book could never have been written.

My very grateful thanks too, to Richard House, the first editor of this series who first suggested the book and helped in its early stages and latterly to Maria Stasiak, the present editor, whose comments during the various stages of production have always led to improvements.

My final thanks are to Jean Reynolds for her wordprocessing and to my wife, Dorothy, for her 'behind the scenes' help in this venture and in all the counselling work I undertake.

1

Why Employ a Counsellor in the Surgery?

In this chapter I first look at the 'traditional' General Practice setting and make some observations about the type of ailments that GPs are asked to help with. I then consider a medical approach which shows awareness of the counselling skills and attitudes that may be used by health professionals. The wisdom of doctors offering lengthy counselling to patients is then discussed along with issues to do with employment of a counsellor in the surgery.

THE GP's APPROACH TO THE PATIENT

'A person, on entering a GP's surgery, is transformed into a patient who is ready to put himself into the hands of the staff and to give up some degree of self-responsibility.' So writes Dr Roger Burford, a GP for over twenty years, when asked to comment on how he sees the situation of the individual who seeks medical help from the surgery. He goes on to say, 'People are trained from a very early age to become patients when they need medical attention. The very word "patient" is descriptive of the attitude required – receptive, long-suffering and non-questioning.'

To this description we might also add the word 'passive', and contrast it with its opposite 'active'. The patient is one who, traditionally, lets things be done to him, does what he is told and looks to the doctor and other medical persons as the experts who should know the answer to his problem and who will restore him to health by the appropriate treatment.

THE GP's PRACTICE AND PERSONNEL

An understanding of the way a General Practice works is invaluable for any counsellor who wishes to work in a doctors' surgery. Dr Burford describes the setting as a complex, ever-changing organisation devoted to the promotion, restoration and maintenance of health, which has three components: the staff, the premises and the patients, the functioning of which are mutually interactive. In describing the staff, he reminds us that there are others as well as the doctors whose position the counsellor must be aware of. He writes:

> Rightly or wrongly, the doctors tend to lead the surgery team. Their training, based on a 'search, find and treat' approach tends to make them directive and authoritative. The all-embracing nature of their contract, together with their exceptional job security, invests them with a power grounded in a permanency not found in many other situations. Their round-the-clock responsibilities and Hippocratic traditions foster and maintain a 'sheepdog-like' jealousy over the welfare of their flock, coupled with a certain degree of self-righteousness. However flawed this system might sound, the blend of power and responsibility, provided that it is tempered with kindness and humour, often produces an effective and economical way of delivering primary health care.
>
> Receptionists have long suffered from 'bad press'. They, like the comedian's mother-in-law, have been the butt of many jokes, and it is not difficult to see the reasons why. Their job is to police the interface between doctors and patients and to try to please both groups at the same time. This is very difficult to do, given the often stressful nature of the work. However, since in most surgeries the receptionists are chosen and employed by the doctors, their attitudes and behaviour will reflect and also be the responsibility of their employers.
>
> Practice nurses are an independent breed. Whilst selected and employed by their doctors, they are professionals who are accustomed to working and making decisions on their own. They have their own professional boundaries which they jealously guard.
>
> The cleaning, gardening and handyman personnel have

an important role in the grooming of the surgery. They are also directly employed by the doctors.

Thus the average surgery workforce, despite its concessions to the 'team approach' is a tight hierarchy with the doctors, as self-employed independent contractors, firmly at its head.

Turning to premises, Dr Burford reminds us that whether they are dilapidated or palatial, they have in common the fact that they are the meeting ground on which health transactions take place, and that for such transactions to take place there are 'ground rules' which existing staff and patients know and which new staff and new patients have to learn. One such 'rule' is the recognition that when a person enters the surgery he is transformed into a patient who is ready to put himself into the hands of the staff and to give up some degree of self-responsibility. The staff, for their part, agree to accept this responsibility and to give it back when the patient leaves the building. The patient, for his part, expects the doctor to be totally concerned with his welfare, up-to-date in his knowledge and to be considerate, kind and always available. In the patient's eyes, thus, the doctor should be perfect; in reality there are about as many perfect doctors as there are patients!

Dr Burford acknowledges flaws in the above approach but maintains that it does produce 'an effective and economical way of delivering primary health care'. As a patient myself who has had far more needs to consult my GP in the last ten years than in the previous fifty, I would agree, and so would very many other people whom I know. The very fact that so many surgeries now have appointments systems shows one way in which the patient's time as well as the doctor's is considered important, and has made for a more equable relationship. The fact that nowadays one is more likely to find a patient in the consulting room sitting at the side of the doctor's desk than with the desk firmly between them, also shows a way in which attitudes towards patients have changed.

So what are the problems that patients bring to their GPs? In general these can be categorised under (1) physical pain, (2) some kind of bodily change which may or may not be painful or (3) some kind of mental and/or emotional worry. The patient expects the doctor as expert to be able to help, and in respect of the first two categories the doctor will usually be able to do so. It is the third category which causes problems for the doctor as well as for the patient. Mental/emotional problems can be treated by physical means, by prescribed drugs which can alleviate symptoms and may be sufficient. But it has been reckoned that one-third of problems that are brought to GPs come under this heading; and, also, that of a GP's time, 25 per cent of patients take up 75 per cent of it!

Furthermore, for years it has been recognised that a number of conditions that appear to be simply physical have a 'mind' component to them – the illnesses known as psychosomatic, which include ulcers and even arthritis. Tension in the mind can lead to changes in bodily behaviour. One of my clients a few years ago traced the beginnings of her long-standing colitis problem to the tensions brought about by the divorce of her parents. All of us are born, it seems, with some areas of our body stronger and other parts weaker. Tension is understandably likely to have its effect on whatever part or parts are weaker; in one person it will be the heart, in another the limbs, in another the stomach, in another the head, etc. Thus even those conditions which seem purely physical may have an emotional aspect to them, due to tension and worry.

In their surgeries nowadays most GPs allow ten minutes for an appointment, and they will often give more time if this is needed. But if there is concern, as there should be, over the causes of a condition as well as the symptoms, it can be doubted whether even fifteen or twenty minutes is sufficient. Thus if the causes of tension, worry and anxiety are to be considered, where there are very often links to the patient's relationships with other people, at home or at work, more time is needed and also the training that enables the right kind of care and concern for problems that have their sources in the emotions and/or in the mind.

It is of course true that in the same way that not all mental and emotional problems need the help of a psychiatrist, so not all of them need the services of a trained counsellor. There is a good reason for doctors and other surgery workers to learn counselling skills. There are courses which are limited to teaching such skills, for short-term work with patients and where there is not the need to give the usual fifty-minute sessions. The understanding and use of such skills may mean, in some instances, that patients will not need to be referred to the trained counsellors, and, in other cases, that the GP will refer patients at an earlier stage than he might otherwise have done. Such skills particularly emphasise empathic listening, showing understanding and acceptance, and becoming aware of the kinds of problems that the health-worker-as-counsellor himself or herself finds it hard to handle, in other words, realising one's limitations.

A MEDICAL APPROACH WHICH SHOWS AWARENESS OF COUNSELLING SKILLS

Dr Burford has described what can be termed the traditional relationship between medical personnel and patients. Both he and other such personnel may in practice view that relationship rather differently. For example, Dr Iain Duncan, another GP, believes the consultation process (sometimes summarised under the mnemonic S-O-A-P: Subjective (history-taking); Objective (clinical findings); Assessment (diagnosis); and Prescription (treatment/management)) is able to be patient-orientated. Thus in history-taking, the doctor can imagine what it feels like to be the patient with this complaint and can show that he understands by his words or his gestures. When proposing to carry out a particularly invasive examination of a patient, he can give the patient the chance to agree or disagree to this, and to express any concerns. He can also indicate to the patient that he (the GP) believes that the patient has control about what others do to his/her body and that he respects that control and the patient in general. In assessing/diagnosing, the doctor can ask the patient what he feels or thinks is wrong with him. This gives the opportunity for fears and fantasies to be voiced and accepted, and where appropriate, repudiated. Many patients, for example, fear they may have cancer, and if the doctor gives them the space to voice such fears themselves, the rapport between patient and doctor is helped. When considering offering a prescription or a way of managing the medical condition, the doctor can ask the patient what he feels like doing in response to the situation and what he feels about the doctor's proposals.

Such a 'patient-centred' approach itself derives from the

work of Carl Rogers, one of the foremost American psychologists of this century, who, working originally in the psychoanalytic tradition of Freud, became dissatisfied with the therapeutic distance between therapist and client which that approach advocated. In the 1940s, Rogers began to use a method which emphasised the relating of counsellor to client in a more personal, open way. For the relationship to succeed and to help the client, Rogers postulated the 'core conditions' of empathic understanding, unconditional positive regard and congruence. Iain Duncan's application of the S-O-A-P process described above shows the influence of empathic understanding in what he says about the history-taking process. In encouraging the patient to voice his feelings, views and concerns during the history-taking and other consultation processes, the doctor can show he is taking the patient seriously as a person and is not being judgemental over what the patient reveals or the doctor observes. This valuing and respecting the patient as an individual is in keeping with Rogers' unconditional positive regard. By 'congruence' Rogers implied honesty and sincerity – the agreement between words spoken and feelings felt. Suppose the doctor feels upset or irritated by something the patient has said. He wants to show 'unconditional positive regard' and accept the patient without being judgemental, but his feelings over what the patient has said are ones of irritation. If the doctor can reflect his own feeling while showing respect for and acceptance of the patient as a person, even if he cannot approve of everything the patient says or does, then he is being congruent for the benefit of the patient, himself and the relationship.

To apply consistently a person-centred approach throughout all the turmoil of General Practice is far from easy for a GP. Iain Duncan admits this but he summarises his position with the following:

I believe that only by trying to apply such an approach can we best help our patients. It should be remembered that at least one-third of patients may present with psychosomatic or overtly emotional problems, and that for all there are the emotional effects of the illness upon the patient to be considered. For many patients the response of a person-centred doctor to the normal components of the medical transaction will be therapeutic enough, and by training and experience doctors can extend their ability to respond, in a counselling mode, to a wide range of emotional problems. But the prevalence and complexity of these, and the need to deal with the physical components of the patient's presentation and the time constraints, mean that frequently the doctor will be glad of the increasing availability of a counselling colleague in the surgery.

TRAINING IN COUNSELLING SKILLS

It is just possible that some health workers are 'natural counsellors', for whom any formal training is unnecessary. But we can ask whether even those who are very sensitive and understanding of others are good at 'looking at their own values, prejudices and other blocks to empathy and good communication'. Veronica Morrell writing on 'Developing counselling skills' (1992: 16) lists that as being integral to a counselling skills course of some twenty-five hours in length spread over ten evenings. Other skills that would be practised as well as discussed would be those of reflecting back and summarising; active listening skills in which the counsellor shows that she has fully understood the client, and enables the client to feel this. Such skills, involving verbal and non-verbal communication, are different from the skills of, say, taking blood from and giving injections to patients. For some doctors and nurses the former, communication skills, may be more difficult than the latter, where the training in correct technique is felt to be more specific. Counselling skills are likely to be learnt more by role-play than by discussion alone and will involve course members taking the part of 'client' as well as 'counsellor' and obtaining feedback from tutors and other course members. Giving time to listening sensitively to someone who has been bereaved by death, or what can be often more painful, by a broken relationship, or to someone who needs to talk over feelings about having been diagnosed as having a crippling illness can be very wearing as well as time-consuming. Health workers' abilities and readiness to help patients with such problems can be helped by counselling skills courses.

Another important feature in such learning is not so much to do with skills as with attitude, especially about feeling happy with being open in one's attitude. Doctors are expected to know the answers. Admitting that one does not know, even to colleagues, can be quite difficult, and it is even more so to patients. But the problems that clients often bring to counsellors are ones where there is a great deal of confusion and many mixed feelings. The counsellor herself feels confused and has to live with that confusion and thereby help the client through it until things become clearer. The attitude the counsellor has to have is one of being ready to live with uncertainty and to admit that uncertainty to colleagues, and to clients when it is appropriate, rather than to dissemble. To live with uncertainty about his patient may not be at all easy for a doctor.

However, even if he has been ready to attend a counselling skills course or indeed a full counselling course and has learnt much about himself and about how to live with uncertainty, a GP will always be up against the problem of time. Let us suppose he does decide to use his counselling skills to help a bereaved patient. A bereavement situation can bring not just tears and grief, but feelings of anger and guilt, to mention but two. And these may be deep-seated in their origins and may have been there for a long time. Thus the genuine tears that accompany the grief over a parent's death may also be punctuated with: '... but I hate her/him for what they did over ... and how my brother/sister always seemed to be the favoured one. ...' However genuine the counselling skills displayed by the empathic doctor, it is going to take time, and possibly a number of counselling sessions, before these complex feelings brought about by a bereavement can be resolved. It is for such a situation that the trained counsellor will be needed. A GP may well find himself in deeper water than he anticipated if he tries to counsel people himself.

If we take the potential and at present mythical client mentioned above who brings her bereavement grief to the GP, but also hints in the first brief interview about her feelings, the GP will note these and realise further time is needed and invite the patient to return, perhaps allocating half-an-hour for the next interview. At that meeting he will perhaps gently remind her what she brought up last time and invite her to say more. The patient may then take up the whole of the half-hour, much of it in tears, going on and on about her early childhood, how her mother never understood her, always seems to be pressurising her, how she would turn to her Dad of whom she was fonder and how he was caught in a dilemma between showing he sympathised with her but felt he must support his wife, etc. The patient is still in full cry when the half-hour ends. Somewhat bemused and pretty exhausted, the GP offers a further half-hour. When he gets home that evening and his wife asks how his day has gone he mentions the interview with this patient. 'That sounds just like my cousin's family' says his wife and immediately the two of them get involved in a lengthy discussion about what happened in that family and what further help he can be to his patient. After an hour they begin to realise the time that has been taken up. 'You are wonderful the way you listen to these patients and really do try to help them', says the wife, 'but is this really your job to help over such involved issues? What about the vicar, shouldn't he be brought in to help?' 'I don't think he is a very good listener', her husband replies. 'Oh, I disagree, he was a great help when Mrs Green's husband died, so I was told', responds the wife. And then there is a further half-hour on the issue of how much help the vicar is.

That sort of scenario shows what can happen once a GP allows himself to become more involved than he really has time for. Nor has he been trained to spend time enabling the client 'to help himself or herself, to clarify difficulties and attempt to resolve them' without 'over-defending' or 'over-identifying', as Nancy Rowland puts it in her chapter on 'Counselling and counselling skills' (1992: 2, 6).

Thus, reluctant though the GP may be to employ a counsellor, there will very likely be problems if he takes too much upon himself. Dr Burford acknowledges that all those who worked in his surgery – doctors, receptionists, nurses – were doing their best to be sympathetic listeners, even creative listeners at times; giving patients a life-line in a time of crises, but admitting that in the end the patients had to swim by themselves or sink. While most of this help tended to be incident-related and of short duration, sometimes a longer time was needed for consultations and then the doctor, as in the example above, might find himself somewhat submerged by the complexities which patients were bringing. As well as the kind of crisis situation brought about by a bereavement which initially might seem to need only a session or two to resolve but which once involvement starts, is seen to be more and more complex, there is a problem of patients who come to the doctor again and again with the same problem which never seems to go away, those who have been described, maybe rather cruelly, as 'heart-sink' patients. As Dr Burford puts it:

> I certainly used to find myself getting bogged down with the same weary workload; patients who week after week seemed to want to rehearse the same story over and over again. Sympathetic listening can be very wearing on the ears, particularly if it does not satisfy a patient's needs.

RELUCTANCE TO EMPLOY A COUNSELLOR

However, it may not be easy for a GP to accept that a counsellor can help the patient more than he can. Dr Burford puts it well as he looks back on the decision which he and his colleagues eventually took: 'Whilst part of me felt interested and excited at the prospect of having a counsellor working with us in the practice, another part of me felt aggressive towards the "intruder" and protective towards my patients.'

Such feelings about intrusiveness and protection may well account for other GPs' reluctance to employ a counsellor, for while a counsellor may be considered just another member of a surgery team, as nurses and receptionists are, in another way a counsellor is not. A counsellor may well be seeing a patient over several, or even many, weeks, for some fifty minutes each time. The material the client brings may well be very personal matters that have not been or may never be brought to the GP, to do with family, work or even treatment at the hands of doctors and other health professionals. It is understandable that a GP may want to know what is going on in these counselling sessions in the same way that, when I was running a counselling course and some of the students wished to work in small groups or in pairs on material that was personal to themselves, I know there was a bit of me that would like to have known what they were discussing. Letting go of one's own feelings of curiosity and protectiveness is not easy. The GP who decides to employ a counsellor will need to do this.

REASONS FOR EMPLOYING A COUNSELLOR IN A SURGERY

There are other very good reasons why a GP should not attempt to offer prolonged counselling times to patients. Their clinical work will suffer if they devote the time normally considered appropriate for a counselling session, thirty to fifty minutes, to some patients regularly; if the GP has the average case-load of about 2,500 patients, as is likely in a city practice, he will find it a considerable intellectual and emotional challenge to try to offer and sustain a relationship of non-possessive warmth (to use another Rogerian term) to all this number and, if he attempts to do it with some, others are likely to suffer. Furthermore, some patients will not want to discuss with their GPs, whom they will be seeing year after year, matters which are very personal. GPs, who often live in the same area as their patients, may well number some of their patients among their personal friends. Counsellors are less likely to live in the area of the practice, will never, if they are wise, take on as clients people they already know, and while they will get to know their clients very well during the period of counselling, will rarely come across them when it ends. The above points are very well made by Rowland *et al.* (1990: 119).

Being able to see a counsellor in a familiar setting, their GP's surgery, will make it easier for some patients to accept counselling. They will be coming to a venue which they know rather than having to journey to one that is unknown. There is also the matter of distance. Before he had a counsellor in his surgery, Dr Burford's patients would be having to make a journey of some twenty-five miles to see a counsellor. He was also aware of his reluctance to refer patients to someone whose character and qualifications were unfamiliar and whom he had never met, whereas when employing his own counsellor he is making a referral to a helper known to him.

He has also found that the counsellor can be an additional resource and support for other members of his primary health care team and that the presence of a counsellor in the surgery can somehow change the atmosphere. In his surgery he feels the approach has become more 'wholesome'; more 'rounded' might be another expression that could be used. He feels he and his colleagues have always been concerned about their patients as people, but he is also aware that since the appointment of the counsellor, it is not just that he and his colleagues have someone they can talk to and offload their feelings occasionally and briefly, but that there has been a growth of understanding and acceptance among all the staff.

The employment of counsellors in surgeries is not new. I first became aware of this when I was a counsellor with the Barnet, Haringey and Hertsmere Marriage Guidance Council (now RELATE), in the 1970s and several of my colleagues were starting to work in surgeries as well as at the Council. Two of these colleagues were married to GPs and had gathered from their husbands that there were patients whom the doctors had recommended to contact the Council, but who were unwilling to do so because this meant contact with and a visit to an unfamiliar setting. Such patients were prepared to see a counsellor in the familiar premises of the surgery. That such schemes were spreading in the 1970s is shown by Heisler (1979), whose research among 150 Marriage Guidance Councils found some 50 surgeries in which Marriage Guidance counsellors worked, involving some 70 counsellors. One of Heisler's conclusions was: 'Most of these schemes are experienced as being very positive both for the counsellors and from the community point of view as a greater variety of clients are seen.' In 1993 it is estimated by RELATE that there are some 150 counsellors and sex therapists working within GP practices, under various contract arrangements.

Another reason why clients may well prefer the familiar setting of the surgery is that the surgery waiting room contains people with a wide variety of problems, including the many physical ones to the admitting of which no stigma is normally attached. Those who visit a specialist agency like RELATE have to accept that they will be seen entering a centre to which people go who have relationship problems. For some this may not be easy. In a surgery they could be there for any number of reasons. There is more anonymity about the setting.

We can now turn to the type of problem over which a doctor may refer patients for counselling. In this connection, an important point has been made by Roger Burford when he says, apropos of the sympathetic listening previously done by himself and his surgery colleagues: 'I believe that our approach to counselling was actually counter-productive, because it medicalised and thus gave illness credibility to problems that were non-medical in origin.'

Many of the problems that clients bring are to do with relationships; broken, failing, unsatisfactory in one way or another; and with their feelings. It is probably these to which Burford refers as non-medical. They are certainly to do with emotions and, even if the symptoms are manifested in seemingly physical conditions like headaches, indigestion, aches and pains in various parts of the body, the cause can be seen as feelings-related rather than body-related.

How well trained are doctors to consider and take note of patients' feelings? As an example I quote the case of a counselling colleague shortly due to have a baby. She had been told the baby would have to be induced and was expecting to go into hospital on a particular day and had, with her husband who had arranged to lighten his work schedule for the days immediately after the birth, made all the necessary preparations for her expected days in hospital. Then a fortnight before the event, she was told the size of the baby was such that it could be born when labour began, which of course could be some days after the date for which she and her family had prepared themselves. At no time did the doctor ask her how she felt about this change of plan. He was the decision-maker – he did not seem to want to know about her feelings. A counsellor, or the doctor who follows the kind of approach advocated by Dr Duncan would surely see the need to ask how the patient feels. Such an enquiry will show the doctor is sensitive and will also help the patient to adjust to the changes that are being suggested and accept them. Maybe, it can be argued, patients should tell their doctors how they feel but it takes a brave patient to say to a doctor, 'How do you think I feel about this?' Thus the emotional difficulties (feelings) will go undetected by staff, a point that Dickson (1989: 361) finds in his research. A simple question about how the patient feels about a course of treatment or a change in the expected treatment is very different from becoming involved in a deeper way with patients' feelings.

Doctors are one of the professional groups at greatest risk

of depression, marital breakdown and suicide (Zigmond 1984, cited in McLeod 1988) and it is unwise for doctors who are unprepared and untrained to take on patients' feelings as well as their medical problems. Yet research has shown that the problems patients bring are often concerned with feelings. For example Hudson (1988) carried out a study of twenty-four GP practices in the Bristol area, and obtained figures which suggested that of the 200,000 patients in the surgeries, over a quarter had a psychological problem and about one-sixth a social one. Only four of the surgeries used the services of a qualified counsellor, though in sixteen the doctors undertook counselling within normal surgery hours. Her analysis of the doctors' comments, however, led her to conclude: 'GPs are inadequately trained for their potential psychological work-load, and it is small wonder that GPs reach for the prescription pad to provide psychotropic drugs.' She recalls how one GP said to her: 'I let a patient talk for a few minutes when I realise their problem is not physical. Then I become aware that time is getting on, so I start writing a prescription.' He went on to say: 'Patients always know that a prescription is the termination of a consultation and automatically stop talking.'

We have thus, from the authors quoted above and from the views in this chapter from Drs Burford and Duncan, good evidence for referral to the trained helper who has the expertise and the understanding, and above all, the time to listen to patients, show understanding and acceptance, and help the alleviation of the pain they are bringing which has a non-physical origin. A case has been made for counselling in GPs' surgeries.

THE TRAINING OF COUNSELLORS WHO WORK IN SURGERIES

Should there be specific rather than only general training for counsellors who are to work in surgeries? A study of twenty-four training institutions to find out what specialist training is given or will be given for counsellors working in primary health care revealed that only one of the nineteen institutions which responded 'had given primary care issues prior thought and had already implemented focussed training provision' (Basharan *et al.* 1992: 13).

The questionnaire they had been sent had been designed after consultations with GPs and counsellors working in the setting. It had identified a number of key areas which should be included in a course for those working in primary health care, such as brief therapy, training in diagnostic skills, collaboration with GPs and other health professionals and various specific topics such as sexual abuse, substance abuse and chronic and terminal illness. However, the respondents to the questionnaire tended not to mention the above areas but instead mentioned those which were felt to be relevant for counsellors working in any setting, including GP practices, such as anxiety, bereavement, depression, phobias, eating disorders, violence, stress management, assertiveness, retirement/redundancy/unemployment. Of the above topics in the questionnaire, sexual and substance abuse were mentioned by the respondents but not the others. However, the mention of these other areas in the questionnaire may prompt training institutions to give them greater prominence in the future.

One of the matters on which there was definite agreement was over the need for supervision. However extensive initial training is, a counsellor is always liable to be faced with problems or situations that 'throw' him. The individual supervisor and/or the supervision group is where any such problems should be brought.

One of the difficulties faced by trainers is the extent to which they should follow their own ideals or be influenced by those outside who suggest they know what the customer wants. For example, because of the demand for counselling in GPs' surgeries, and to cut down waiting lists, it may seem right to suggest that trainees are informed about and given practice in 'brief therapy'. However, the training institution of the person-centred tradition might feel that therapy should continue for as long as client and counsellor feel it is helpful. To encourage brief therapy (whatever 'brief' may mean) would be to compromise the institution's ideals because 'we don't pay attention to issues regarding the number of sessions we give our clients' (Basharan *et al.* 1992: 11). The researchers concluded their report by saying, 'The majority expressed an interest in exploring the subject further, perhaps in the form of a working party which ... might eventually draw up some general training guidelines' (13). The organisation which carried out this research, the Counselling in Primary Care Trust, has plans to get 8,000 accredited counsellors to work full-time in GPs' surgeries, and it is thus possible that if more and more counsellors are employed there, training institutions will adapt to further needs that are highlighted.

DISCUSSION ISSUES

1 Think of visits you have made to GPs. What, in your experience, are the ingredients for a satisfactory/unsatisfactory consultation?
2 Do you think that talking about what seems to be a physical illness can help?
3 Have you ever found yourself over-involved in someone's problems?

2

The Referral of Patients for Counselling

The types of problems which clients bring is first considered and the problem of depression is discussed briefly. Having looked at the decision the GP has to make as to whether the patient should be referred for counselling or for psychiatric help, I then deal with the referral process and resistance to counselling, with examples of how this has been overcome. I then consider how subsequent appointments are best made and the kinds of situation that require the counsellor to have contact with the GP. Liaison with other members of the surgery team is then looked at and the chapter concludes with a section on confidentiality.

WHICH PATIENTS COME FOR COUNSELLING IN A SURGERY?

The patients whom a GP recommends for counselling may be having relationship problems: maybe with a spouse, maybe with a partner of the same or opposite sex, maybe with a parent or offspring; or may be experiencing misery because of the difficulty of forming any close relationship; or may be relating on the surface perfectly well to family and to work colleagues but, while outwardly apparently confident, feel inwardly insecure and fearful; or may be suffering from panic attacks or some unaccountable anxiety; or may be depressed because of an accident or a physical illness; or may be in a job where there is much stress; or may be out of a job and feeling useless; or may have been subject to some abuse years ago and now feel more bothered by this than in the immediate

17

past, possibly because of the way abuse has been given much more publicity in the media these last few years. In all such problems it is the emotions and the feelings that are affected.

The pain that is felt when emotions are affected is usually less easy to treat than when the pain or discomfort is in a particular part of the body. Even if the symptoms can be helped by anti-depressant drugs or minor tranquillisers, the causes ideally need to be brought out and worked through. For example, the current problems with a partner may well be linked to the relationship with one or both parents; the depression may be due to having felt the need to repress all feelings of anger for many years. Feelings of guilt, feelings over having felt let down on one or many occasions, feelings of inadequacy and of low self-esteem – these are very common in the clients who come for surgery counselling. Helping them takes considerable time. Even thirty hours of counselling is a very short time when so many of the problems that are brought go back many years.

Depression is a problem that clients frequently bring to their counsellors and may at times be very difficult to deal with. Sometimes the reasons for it seem very clear to both counsellor and client – the depression has arisen because one or more events have led to it. This kind of depression is known as reactive. It is easier to help a client over this kind of depression than over the kind known as endogenous, which comes from within the client, as it were, and has not been caused only by events which the client found it very hard to cope with. Doctors themselves as well as counsellors may differ over how much even that depression results from life events, especially those which occurred very early in life, the memory of which has been suppressed. But it is very important that all of us recognise that such depression may have a biochemical cause and that further research may show that there is some chemical imbalance in the brain that can be righted by medication.

Some patients with depression may experience mood swings, a condition known as manic depression. When they are 'up' they certainly do not want counselling – they feel fine. When they are 'down' equally they do not want counselling – they feel so down they could not even get to the surgery, let alone talk about their condition. It can be difficult, therefore, for these patients to accept counselling.

The distinction between endogenous and reactive depression itself is not absolute. They can coexist in the same person and indeed it would be very rare for the person who has had episodes of endogenous depression not to suffer from reactive depression because the fall in mood due to the imbalance of brain chemicals, if sustained, will make the sufferer incapable of making the best life decisions. As a result of this, relationships, work and family life will all suffer.

REFERRAL TO A COUNSELLOR OR TO ANOTHER SPECIALIST?

The areas of problems in which counsellors work are more akin to those of the clinical psychologist or psychiatrist than those of the consultant physician or surgeon. Psychology and psychiatry are the two disciplines which provide the material used in counsellor training rather than any of the other medical specialities.

Thus one of the decisions the GP has to make is whether to refer to a counsellor or to one of these other two specialities, the clinical psychologist or psychiatrist.

Those patients who are so very severely depressed that they could never take the initiative to try to make an appointment themselves; those who suffer from severe obsessions and compulsions; those who are so psychotic that they feel, in their paranoia, that everyone else is to blame other than themselves; those whose thinking and speech are so bizarre that they are no longer properly in contact with what the vast majority feel is the real world; all these will clearly be referred for psychiatric help, or to a clinical psychologist, where it is felt that behavioural changes can be brought about by means other than simply medication. Counsellors are trained to work with people who, temporarily, are experiencing more unhappiness or more of a sense of isolation than is customary for most people at some period of their lives. If we have very understanding parents, relatives and friends we will probably be able to work through such distresses on our own without further help. Other means by which people may tend to cope with distress is by recourse to alcohol, tobacco or non-prescribed drugs. Dependency on such substances has traditionally seemed more acceptable than taking up the time of another person. It may well be more recognised now that accepting the need for counselling and thus, for a time, some dependency on the relationship with a professional helper, shows more maturity than denying the need for that kind of dependency, but allowing dependency on substances.

Another group of patients who may be referred for counselling are those who would like to see a psychiatrist but are non-urgent cases and who are thus unlikely to get an appointment for some months. The GP may suggest to them that they seek counselling as an interim measure, to help them over the following weeks until their appointment comes through. The psychiatrist may then take them on him or herself, or recommend that they continue with their counselling, because there are no signs of present or incipient mental illness.

In contrast to this latter group, there are those who firmly do not want to be referred to a psychiatrist because such a referral will be on their medical records and might have to be revealed to a potential employer or training course leader. A note on their records that they have seen a counsellor will not, they feel, carry the same stigma; this was noted by MacLeod (1988: 11) in her research among fourteen General Practices.

THE REFERRAL PROCESS AND MAKING APPOINTMENTS

Having decided that referral to the counsellor in the surgery is more appropriate than to a psychiatrist, how should the GP arrange this?

Discussion with several colleagues working in other surgeries to which they are attached as members of the surgery team indicates that the message conveyed to the patient by the GP is somewhat like this:

> From what you have told me, I believe you could be helped by the counsellor we have working here. The counsellor will be able to offer you much more time than I can and has been trained to listen to people and to help them work out solutions to the problems they are bringing. I will let our counsellor know that I am referring you and the counsellor will be in touch with you when she is able to give you an appointment.

Such a message gives the patient little choice in the matter. The GP is saying that the patient should see the counsellor and it is very difficult for the patient to refuse. The next procedure is for the GP to notify the counsellor that the patient has been recommended for counselling, either, for example, by writing the patient's name, address and phone number in the counselling referral book or by informing the counsellor of these details direct. Some doctors insist on writing a referral letter, as they would to any medical specialist, such as a consultant, and, as one counselling colleague said to me, such a letter may be helpful not only to the counsellor, but for the GP himself, as the very act of writing will help the GP to clarify his own thinking about the patient and the problem.

Whether the referral is by a note in a book, a note to the counsellor or by means of a full referral letter, the next stage is for the counsellor to contact the client when an appointment becomes available, or for the receptionist to make the contact. De Groot (1985) in a survey among forty-six Marriage Guidance Councils which employed a counsellor, found that fifty-one out of seventy-four counsellors said that the receptionist made the initial appointment. In eighteen cases the counsellor was given the patient's phone number and made the appointment himself.

There are distinct advantages in the procedure in which the counsellor makes the appointment. The client is hearing from the actual person who is going to see them and thus feels the contact to be more personal. Further, many clients are at work in the daytime or out of their homes shopping, etc., and receptionists on the whole will not be in a position to phone in the evenings. The counsellors I have spoken to are able and willing to do this. Although De Groot's research shows that the majority of appointments were made by receptionists, this may not be the preferred procedure for either counsellors or potential clients.

In the referral procedures so far discussed, the patient has not been required to take any initiative to obtain counselling. The doctor has recommended, the counsellor or receptionist has been informed and contact is made. The patient can, of course, refuse the appointment or simply not turn up, but the initiative has been taken by others.

My own preference is for the doctor to recommend counselling, to give the patient a short leaflet about it, and for the patient then to decide whether he or she wants an

appointment, by telling the receptionist or whoever is responsible for appointments. It is the patient who is thus making the
final decision and is being an active agent in the process.
Counselling is very different from medical procedures where
the patient is being 'done to', is being examined by the specialist, is being x-rayed, is having a tooth taken out or part of the
body massaged. In counselling, the patient is having to
express, having to think, having to look at himself and reassess, as well as being helped to feel a worthwhile person. As
it is an active process from the patient's point of view, so, I
feel, it is of importance for the patients to take even the slight
initiative of indicating that they wish or are prepared to accept
counselling.

RESISTANCE TO SEEING A COUNSELLOR

Among some patients, there is still a tendency to equate
emotional problems with mental ones and to feel that anyone
seeking help over these must be 'going mad'. These patients
may well feel that seeing a counsellor is like having to see a
psychiatrist and that if they have to see the former, this is, as
it were, the first step on a ladder that will lead as a second
step to seeing a psychiatrist and hence to being considered a
'mental case'. If they have these fears, it is to be hoped that
their GP can discover this from them and reassure them.

Others feel that emotional problems should be 'kept in the
family'. They may indicate to their GP that all is not well with
their relationships, but may not be willing to expound further,
either to him or to anyone else. Such patients may take a lot
of convincing that counselling can help them.

Then there are those people who pride themselves on being
'copers'. These are often professional people like nurses and
church leaders whose job it is to help others and who feel it is
an admission of defeat to have to seek help over emotional
as compared with physical problems. With these patients Dr
Burford uses a 'softly softly' approach, suggesting they return
to see himself for two or three further appointments, so that
he can introduce the idea of counselling to them gradually. He
takes time, in other words, to help them to see that counselling
could be of help to them. As he says himself:

If it were a hernia they were bringing me, I need only five minutes to recommend that they see a surgeon with a view to an operation. It will take very many more minutes to come to the point where I can suggest they try counselling.

Other patients may believe that 'just talking cannot possibly help', and/or that they themselves could be terribly embarrassed because 'I just shan't know what to say'. Geraldine was recommended by her GP to see a counsellor, but she was not at all keen. However, she did agree to come fortnightly, though she ended each interview by saying, 'How can all this talking help?' The time arrived for the counsellor's summer break and this was talked through during the preceding interviews; the client appeared to understand that there would be a break of four weeks.

She did not turn up for her appointment immediately before the break, but came instead the following week when the counsellor had already started her holiday. She waited at the surgery for some time and then went home. When she next saw her GP and he asked her about the counselling, she said she was very angry and that the counsellor had broken the appointment. On the counsellor's return from holiday the GP told her what had happened and suggested she get in touch with the client. She did so and the client resumed counselling, and seemed in a much more co-operative frame of mind. Perhaps the explanation for her change of heart was that the client had realised she had made a mistake over the dates and that the counsellor had 'forgiven' her.

Matilda, a counsellor, had a client who came very reluctantly for counselling, for whom a very gentle and patient approach was needed. This patient had been told by the GP that counselling would help in bringing down his high blood pressure, but when he came he was very sceptical. Matilda allowed him to tell his story in a very chatty, informal way, as he might to a friend in a pub, rather than in a formal setting. The client talked in what might have seemed a very superficial way and was allowed to do so because Matilda felt that to try to push him to get in touch with deeper feelings would simply drive him away from counselling. Very gradually over some five fortnightly interviews he did get in touch with his emotions by allowing some of his feelings to be expressed. This enabled him to stand back and see his problems and himself in perspective. What had been mountains became molehills. To assist in this process Matilda used a metaphor which was appropriate for this client in view of the work he did: 'You are between security and prison, letting things come out gradually rather than in a mass break-out.' Such a statement from the counsellor made sense to this client. The outcome was blood pressure greatly reduced, coming off pills and a return to work. In this case the crucial thing seems to have been the gentle approach of the counsellor, letting the client tell the story in a matter-of-fact superficial away, which gradually enabled him to get in touch with feelings.

Resistance can also show itself in other ways, for example in the client who outwardly is quite happy to come for counselling but, when there, seems to the counsellor to be putting on a kind of false protective smile and/or talks very fast and covers many problem areas but resists the counsellor's attempts to get her to focus on any one area. Anthea had one such client whom she discussed in supervision. She spoke of how this client had never seemed to allow anyone to get close to her and seemed to keep everyone at arm's length. The supervisor suggested that the fast talking and refusal to focus was the client's way of keeping the counsellor at a distance. If the counsellor was able to refer to this, to what she felt was happening to herself in the interviews, at least this problem that the client was showing could be looked at more closely and perhaps the reasons why other people had to be kept at a distance could become clearer.

Breaking down resistance to coming for counselling may take various forms, depending on the individuals concerned. James used persuasion in a very directive way when he and a colleague felt that a family session attended by both parents was essential to try to help a long-standing client in whose family there was a lot of love but also a good deal of misunderstanding. When told on the phone that one of the parents was opposed to coming, he stressed how important it was for both to attend as both were important members of the family. It was unclear until the day whether both would attend, but in the event they did and the parent who was said to have been resistant was indistinguishable from the other in this respect. James had to wonder whether the parent who was said to be so resistant was in a sense acting on behalf of the other parent who appeared less resistant but inwardly may have been more so. The parents continued to come for the family sessions.

Earlier in this section I referred to Dr Burford's statement that sometimes he has to spend some considerable time working with a potential client for counselling before he feels they will accept this. It is possible that not all GPs find they do give up that amount of time, but refer patients more hastily. Because the doctor is recommending help from another specialist, such patients feel they must be obedient, but they see counselling as a process by which they will be cured by a specialist. As my colleague Richard House puts it: 'Such an attitude towards counselling fosters or reinforces an attitude or ethos of dependence which is the very antithesis of the personal-responsibility focus to counselling to which I am personally committed' (personal communication). Unless patients are prepared to accept responsibility not only for the changes that they feel they want in their lives but also for the need to go into painful areas themselves in order for those changes to be realised, they may easily either leave counselling after just one or two sessions or remain static during the sessions by repeating the same kind of story week after week and/or talking at a great rate, as Anthea's client did, and eventually leave counselling feeling disillusioned that it 'didn't really help'. For such clients, very careful handling is needed in that the counsellor has to be very sensitive about their resistance and the pain they dare not face while as gently as possible helping them to face the areas that are painful. Richard recalls such a case where there was strong resistance initially but gradually and over a total of fourteen sessions 'the work the client did was truly life-transforming in nature'.

Resistance to counselling, thus, will not be overcome by all the clients that GPs recommend, but provided the GP has prepared his patients for counselling and provided the counsellor is prepared to proceed sensitively, some of those who are initially very resistant will eventually be very glad that they and their counsellor persisted.

MAKING SUBSEQUENT APPOINTMENTS

Having broken down resistance, if there has been any, and having explained to the client that counselling problems are rarely solved in just one or two interviews, the counsellor will then offer a second appointment or a series of appointments. Some counsellors like to make a specific contract for, say, six appointments, with a review at the end and discussion whether to continue; others prefer not to make such a contract, but to make each subsequent appointment at the conclusion of the last, the usual procedure being for the clients to be seen at the same time each week. Whichever procedure is adopted, it is best that subsequent appointments are arranged between counsellor and client and entered by the counsellor in the appointments book.

CONTACT BETWEEN COUNSELLOR AND GP

Some GPs offer the counsellor full access to the patient's notes; counsellors are likely to enter on the notes simply the dates on which they have seen the patient, though periodic remarks such as 'seems much better' or 'counselling seems likely to continue for some time' are also appropriate. Counsellors do not write on such notes any details of what has been discussed.

However, sometimes a counsellor may feel very concerned about a patient, for example, when the patient has talked of suicide, or where there is danger to the patient from someone else or where the patient could be a danger to another.

It is particularly important that GP and counsellor talk with each other when a patient who has been counselled does commit suicide. Sharing the sadness which both feel is important, but also the 'if onlys' which both may be struggling with − 'If only I had not mentioned *that* when talking with the patient when she saw me last', which the counsellor may be thinking and 'If only I had not prescribed that medication', which might be the thought in the doctor's mind. Such thoughts need to be shared and the feelings of guilt and, maybe, the unconscious wish to find someone else to blame need to be brought out between doctor and counsellor and anyone else in the surgery who has been affected by what has happened.

Another example where the counsellor felt the GP should be contacted was over a patient who was very angry with the doctor for not telling him that his wife had a terminal illness. A rather different reason for contacting the GP was over a patient who had been bereaved and where the GP felt the patient would never get over this. The counsellor was able to reassure the GP, having talked with the client at some depth.

Further contact may be necessary because many of the problems that people bring to counsellors in surgeries have a physical aspect to them: headaches, hyperventilating, pains in various parts of their bodies, etc. Both counsellor and doctor may be convinced that the problem lies in the area of mind, spirit, personality – the non-physical – but even so the pains and aches are real enough. Thus Jackie feels that it is appropriate at times to suggest that her client sees the GP again for a further check-up. In a way this may be a bit like 'mother' (herself – a parent) suggesting the client has a further talk with 'father' (the GP), but it also gives the opportunity for the GP to check again whether the symptoms are medical rather than psychosomatic.

However, such referral back to the GP should only be done after due consideration. Counsellors will hope to see their clients improving, but have to acknowledge that sometimes clients remain on a plateau, as it were, for many weeks. Counselling is then very much a 'holding operation', staying with the client through weeks of uncertainty, confusion, struggle. When there are physical symptoms constantly being mentioned by the client, the counsellor may feel under pressure to refer the client back to the doctor. The decision whether or not to do so will depend, after consultation with the GP, on the extent to which both agree the client's apparent physical problem is really 'in the mind'. On the other hand, there is nothing to prevent a client of her own accord going to see her GP whenever she wishes.

Such contact between counsellor and GP may be via a written note or via a short discussion after or even during surgery times. The counsellors in surgeries whom I interviewed have all spoken of their GPs' genuine caring attitude towards their patients and thus readiness to talk about them and to be telephoned at home if necessary.

Contact can also be made more formally via the regular

practice meeting for staff which a number of surgeries have. Matilda, who counsels in three practices, is invited to attend the twice-monthly meeting in one of them. She finds it particularly valuable to be thus seen as a member of the surgery team and to be involved in the discussions about policy and patients. She could not help but contrast this surgery with another where she was not even informed about the appointment of a second counsellor to the practice.

The impression I have got from talking to colleagues in other surgeries has given credibility to the procedure in the surgery where I counsel, that having referred patients to a counsellor, GPs trust the counsellor to work professionally and to consult them when the counsellor has need to do so. Even those doctors who prefer to write a formal referral letter do not expect from counsellors the kind of reply full of medical detail which they will get from medical specialists to whom they refer.

However, it should be noted that the authors of the British Association for Counselling's booklet (Rowland and Hurd 1991: 5, 6) do advocate close liaison between counsellors and GPs. Such advocacy is understandable because of fear of the possibility that a patient might be affected adversely by counselling and the counsellor in a practice, like any other professional, could be sued; also, as a member of the surgery team, the counsellor works under the GP. However, perhaps what is more important than formal written contact is the facilitating atmosphere in a surgery whereby members of the team such as counsellors can feel able to consult the GP when there is need and there is mutual confidence in the different members.

It is also very helpful when counsellor and GP can get to know the general way in which each other work. The counsellor may be providing a service for several GPs in a practice and can become aware of the individual differences in the way they see their job and the way they work with patients, all of which may be perfectly valid. For example Dr Alistair may be very anxious to know how the patients he refers are getting on with the counsellor. He can of course get feedback from the patients themselves when they next see him, but, now that they are seeing the counsellor, this may not be for some weeks. So he will be inclined to ask the counsellor and she feels it entirely right to respond, not breaking the confidentiality by talking about the material the patient has brought, but saying a bit about how she feels about the patient, how the patient seems to be reacting to counselling and in general how things are going. Dr Angus, on the other hand, will not be so curious. He is very professional and once he has handed a patient over to a specialist, he is perfectly content to leave the patient in the specialist's hands until such time as the patient returns to him or he gets a formal letter from the specialist. So he will not be curious about how the counselling is going and will not seek contact with the counsellor. In his way he is as caring and concerned about his patients as Dr Alistair, but he sees the whole matter of referral rather differently. The counsellor in the surgery has herself to recognise the different approaches of the members of the surgery, including, of course the practice nurse who will be entrusted with much of the routine medical work and may also be seeing patients who are being counselled, for blood pressure tests and blood samples, for example.

CONTACT WITH OTHER SURGERY STAFF

There is evidence that ancillary staff in a surgery can be considerably helped by meetings with the surgery counsellor. For example, Christine Garlton, a receptionist, writes how she and her receptionist colleagues were helped to cope better with bereaved patients, with aggressive patients and with drug addicts after they had had an hour-long meeting with the surgery counsellor to look at stress (1992: 35). The temptation to retaliate when someone was aggressive was looked at and alternative responses considered, one of the crucial factors being the receptionist's need to look at her own feelings and body language in such situations. The GPs themselves were also helped by the counsellor, Kay Farquarson, and by the community psychiatric nurse and the psychologist who ran a workshop with the purpose of looking at various consulting styles. The workshop leaders demonstrated the styles and the GPs took the part of patients. Commenting on the effectiveness of such workshops and other less formal meetings one of the GPs commented 'Kay has broadened our thinking and made us, we feel, more empathetic and active listeners to our patients'.

For a counsellor to feel and to be considered by other surgery staff as a member of the practice team, some kind of induction scheme is desirable. This can take the form of the counsellor spending time with each of the other members of the team in which she explains the way she works and hears from them how they work. This will enable a clear understanding of each other's roles and also give a clearer idea of referral possibilities. Time spent with the medical staff will also help the counsellor to have a better understanding of treatment procedures, particularly the effects of psychotropic drugs, points well made by Irving (1992: 28).

Most, if not all, practices now have a practice manager, an administrator who supervises the running of the practice and liaises with the Family Health Services Authority which is responsible for payment of staff.

A counsellor may have more contact with the practice manager than with the GPs, as will probably all ancillary staff in a surgery. My own and other counsellors' experience of working with the practice manager has been a good one, but one counselling colleague, Matilda, had to cope with the following difficulty. She found the practice manager cold, distant and authoritarian. She found she was reacting in a similar way as she had done to some teachers at school when she was 15. She was overawed, fearful and also angry at being treated, she felt, as an inferior rather than as an equal. She was not being taken seriously, the practice manager was not hearing her. She coped with the problem by taking it to supervision and realising the connection between her present feelings and those she had had when she was young. She had to tell herself: 'You are no longer 15; you do not have to react to this man as if you were.' While the relationship problem between herself and the practice manager has not been resolved, she has learnt, through supervision and her own message to herself, to cope with her feelings.

WHEN MIGHT A GP BECOME WORRIED ABOUT A COUNSELLOR'S EFFECTIVENESS?

One of the factors that a counsellor himself should be concerned about is whether clients come back or not. If I saw six new clients and I had arranged a subsequent appointment for all six which seemingly they had accepted and the next week only three of them came a second time and the other three had not contacted us, I should be seriously worried! Similarly, a GP should be concerned if clients seem to terminate counselling early for no good reason. The number of times clients come should range from one interview to around fifteen and some will want to come for many more than that, but if the GP gets feedback from patients that they did not find the counselling helpful, he has to be concerned, especially if he is employing two counsellors and clients stay with the other counsellor for longer and always give him good feedback. The GP would need to talk with the counsellor and try to find reasons. The counsellor should of course be discussing the problem with her supervisor. One of the reasons why things are not going well in the counselling could be changes in the counsellor's own life, maybe the emergence of difficulties over which the counsellor needs to seek the help not just of her supervisor but of a therapist who will give regular therapy for a time. During the period of therapy it may be wiser to give up counselling entirely. The GP himself may have to advise this if he continues to be concerned about how the counsellor is getting on with his patients.

Where there is more than one counsellor working in the same surgery, it is hoped they will meet with each other and share matters of common concern such as how things are going with their clients and whether they are conscious of any 'sibling rivalry' which may exist between themselves.

CONFIDENTIALITY

Even when patients have been referred by their GP, the counsellor should respect confidentiality, which is why any mention on the patient's medical notes will be very general and will not contain material that the client has told the counsellor. Ideally, where the counsellor wants to talk about the patient to the GP or to a consultant or other professional such as a nurse or social worker, she will first ask the patient's permission to do this. However, there may be the occasional instance where the counsellor feels, for reasons of safety and danger, that she is entitled to forgo asking permission. Such a situation may be when the counsellor feels there is a danger of suicide or of the client being violent or if the client is behaving or talking in a very bizarre fashion. The major consideration is what is ultimately in the client's best interest. If the counsellor judges that it is in the patient's best interest that confidentiality be broken, then it is right to break it.

However, such examples are rare. Confidentiality is vitally important because it is not uncommon for clients to tell their counsellors very personal matters that they have never mentioned to anyone else. It is unlikely they will feel safe to do this until they have seen the counsellor several times and feel complete trust. What will take one client a long time to bring out may take another client only a few moments. For example, I recall many years ago two clients who mentioned having had abortions. It took one of them some eight sessions before she was able to refer to this. Another client I was seeing at about the same time mentioned having had an abortion in the first interview. It took her longer to tell of another experience she had had which for her was far more traumatic, her feelings when her mother told her she was going to the shops and in fact was leaving to go to another country. The building up of trust takes time, which is one of the reasons why counsellors ideally should be able to offer weekly appointments of about fifty minutes, at least in the first weeks of counselling. The pressure on the time of most workers in the statutory agencies such as psychiatric and social work makes it very hard for them to give their clients that amount of time and thus, sometimes, to win their confidence.

DISCUSSION ISSUES

1 Have you ever been depressed? What was the response of friends, family or doctor? Were any of the responses helpful?
2 How can patients be helped to accept counselling if they are resistant?
3 Why is teamwork relevant to counselling in a GPs' surgery?

3

Practical Considerations

In this chapter I look first at medication, and at the question of whether the client's being on prescribed drugs interferes with the counselling process. I then discuss practical considerations such as the room used for counselling, furniture, lighting and continuity, as well as whether payment for counselling is part of the therapeutic process. The chapter ends with a look at time-limited counselling and the pressure on counsellors to extend their workload and suggests strategies to deal with these pressures.

TO PRESCRIBE OR NOT TO PRESCRIBE

The drugs that GPs are likely to prescribe for patients who come for counselling are of two types: drugs that are given to relieve anxiety and to enable sleep, and drugs that are given for depression. The first kind are known as hypnotics/anxiolytics (hypnotics so called from the Greek word for sleep: anxiolytics, from words meaning freeing from anxiety). These are used for sedation or for management of acute stress/anxiety/panic/grief reactions. They are likely to be prescribed after, for example, a bereavement or some other shock which leads to sleeplessness and acute anxiety. The best known of them to the lay person is probably Valium (Diazepam). Others in this group are Mogadon, Dalmane and Temazepam and the group as a whole is called benzodiazepines. The Committee on Safety of Medicines has stated that these should only be used for short-term relief (two to four weeks) of severe anxiety and insomnia. However in practice they are sometimes prescribed for emotional distress, relationship difficulties and depression and thus are used long-term rather than short-term. If these drugs are used over a long period, there is a greater chance of some of the twenty physical and fourteen psychological side-effects occurring, such as headaches, blurred vision, impotence, lethargy, agoraphobia, confusion and irritability (Hammersley and Beeley 1992: 162). These authors quote other research which suggests that if these drugs are taken for longer than six months, patients may find it hard to think constructively and may feel they cannot do without the drug.

The second group are the anti-depressants which themselves divide into two kinds, those which have a sedating function and those which are non-sedative. A common one of the first group is Amitriptyline (Tryptizol) and among the non-sedative type are Imipramine (Tofranil) and Clomipramine (Anafranil). Patients who are complaining of sleeplessness are likely to be prescribed one of the sedative type. These drugs take two to three weeks to have any effect on mood, though those that have a sedative function should help over sleep from the beginning. However, there are side-effects such as dry mouth, increased appetite/weight gain, nausea and confusion. There are, in fact, a huge variety of drugs for this condition, including some very expensive ones where side-effects are less pronounced. Anti-depressants are much less likely to cause dependence than the anxiolytics, and withdrawal is not generally characterised by disabling symptoms.

Counsellors vary in their views over whether anxiolytics and anti-depressants are likely to affect counselling. Hammersley and Beeley, in their article 'The effects of medication on counselling' feel that counselling and drugs are incompatible because 'One implicit assumption in counselling is that the client has internal resources to take responsibility for finding real solutions' (1992: 162). Even if clients are on anti-depressants when they come for counselling, these authors feel that they should be gradually withdrawn before counselling ceases in order that material which has been repressed can be given the chance to come out. Counsellors must be aware that sometimes 'stuckness' in the counselling could be due to drugs and could resolve when drugs are reduced or stopped. Ideally they should discuss with the prescriber. A colleague, Simon, who finds that most of his clients are on prescribed drugs when they first come to him, discusses with them ways to reduce their medication and finally come off, after the clients have the GP's consent for this.

He works in a surgery where he always gets a referral letter from the GP and the letter will give details of any medication the patient is having. He finds his main contact with GPs is over this. For example, one of his clients, after much hospitalisation, was on so much medication that he felt she could not possibly benefit from counselling, her perceptions and thinking being so muddled. He discussed this with the doctor and the dose was gradually reduced to a sixth of what had originally been prescribed at the hospital; within three months the patient was able to return to work. Clients who are sedated cannot easily give time and thought to working out with the counsellor how they can deal with their problems. If they are to have counselling and gain from it, dosage has to be reduced to the point where they are able to think and to remember normally. Another counsellor feels that being on certain drugs may mean clients are not as alert as they should be and are inclined to forget what has been said. Thus the counsellor has to go over things with them much more slowly than usual.

Other counsellors report that they are not aware of medication interfering with the counselling but that, nevertheless, it is useful to discuss coming off medication with clients. Clients may not, after all, realise what the real world is like until they do so; for example, one client was advised to come off her drugs gradually before the birth of her child. Having done so, she told the counsellor that she had 'discovered herself', after living for some eight or nine years 'in a haze'.

Sometimes one finds a client who seems over-resistant to taking medication. In this kind of case it may well be appropriate for the counsellor to remind the client that medication can actually help.

Another question that can be asked about medication is whether any interference with the counselling process will depend on the theoretical orientation of the counsellor. It has been suggested that counsellors who adopt a cognitive approach or a behavioural one will be less concerned with the effects of prescribed drugs than a counsellor who emphasises the need for the release of feelings. Counsellors who work more through thinking or who believe that if behaviour can be changed, so will attitude and thinking change, will be concerned that a client's own ability to perceive and think are unimpaired by medication, but will be less concerned if the effect of the drug is to block off feelings of depression and anxiety; whereas the counsellor who feels sure that the important issue is for the client to be able to express feelings, even if painful, and fully experience her or himself at a feeling level, will be concerned if the medication that the client is taking inhibits this process. Medication which is designed to suppress worry and anxiety may make it difficult for the client to express feelings of fear, anxiety and anger.

Whatever different counsellors and researchers believe about the effects of drugs, drugs alone will not help over the causes of the problem that have brought the patient to the doctor. They may alleviate symptoms, help the patient to feel less depressed and to sleep better. Thus they may help to enable a client to remain at work and to make the weekly journey to see the counsellor, as in the case of John.

John had gone to university full of hope that this was to be the happiest time of his life. The reality for him turned out to be very different. He decided he had to leave and he felt a failure. This made him depressed. As well as giving him anti-depressants, his GP recommended counselling and he was able to look not only at why he had found life at that particular university unacceptable, but at the way in general he related to people. Counselling helped him to look in some detail at his life, to reassess it and to think differently about people. For him both the medication and the counselling seemed appropriate and helpful.

As already stated, anti-depressants usually take some time to have an effect. The patient has to persevere with them for some six weeks before any reduction in dosage is considered advisable. Mabel, who was receiving counselling as well as anti-depressants, reported that she was feeling better after some four weeks of the former. She also reported to her doctor that she was putting on weight, and asked if her dosage could be reduced. She told her counsellor that the doctor asked her to continue with the same dosage because the medication could not yet have had any good effect. Her doctor may have recommended counselling, but does not appear to have felt that it could help the depression! In this instance, ideally, the counsellor should have asked the client's permission to discuss the case with the GP. In the event, Mabel herself took the initiative over her medication and took half the prescribed dose. By insisting on the original full dosage being maintained and seemingly not having heard the patient's report that she was feeling better, the GP appeared to be taking a rather different line from that advocated in Chapter 1, where what the patient feels and says should be taken seriously by the doctor.

Another problem that can arise over medication is when the counsellor is made aware that GPs differ among themselves over what is appropriate. Mildred had been on a high dosage of her medication for some years. Then she moved house and her new GP would not prescribe such a high dosage, though apparently she had no side-effects that she was aware of. She contacted our counselling agency in some distress. I realised that she was now in the catchment area of the GPs in whose surgery our agency is located and I mentioned her predicament to the senior GP who agreed to take her on if she wished to transfer. This Mildred did, and her medication was restored to the dosage with which she felt she could face things.

She also came for counselling for some weeks and worked through a number of long-standing problems. During this period, on one occasion she came to the surgery for a renewed prescription and saw one of the other doctors, who also was keen to reduce her dosage. This put her into a panic. When she saw me I felt all I could recommend was that in future she saw her own GP, with whom she was registered. Discussion with this GP led to her very, very gradually reducing her dosage. In this instance, the patient's feelings were taken into account by the GP, and together they agreed on a way of dealing with the medication. Another way which I as the counsellor could have tried to help over the situation would have been to have tried to discuss her medication with both the GPs whom she had seen. I felt it was more satisfactory to suggest to the patient that she made appointments in future with the GP of her choice rather than for me to become involved in the differing viewpoints of the doctors concerned. I gave the patient the opportunity to solve this particular problem her way.

THE PHYSICAL SETTING FOR A COUNSELLING INTERVIEW

The room and the setting

Ideally a room for counselling should be sound-proof, should measure about twelve square feet and should contain two easy chairs, a settee and two upright chairs. It is often assumed that easy chairs are a *sine qua non* for counselling, but sometimes one does have a client who prefers to sit in an upright chair. A settee can be useful if one is counselling a couple. If they are given a choice of where they wish to sit, it can be of some significance if they choose to sit together on the settee or if they both choose the separate chairs, leaving the counsellor to choose between the settee and the uprights. The couple who sit together on the settee may choose this as a means of mutual protection and closeness in the face of this stranger whom they are meeting for the first time. The couple who choose the separate easy chairs may be asserting each in their own way something about independence, particularly if they refrain from asking the counsellor 'Which is your seat?' A settee can be useful in counselling a couple; as a counsellor in that situation I have occasionally invited the couple to sit on it and express how they feel about such greater closeness.

However, it is unlikely that a GPs' surgery will have a room where there is such choice. It is quite possible that the only chairs may be upright ones with hard rather than soft seats, and the room may have a medical couch in it rather than any armchairs or settees. How much does this really matter?

It probably does matter if the counsellor has been led to believe during training that easy chairs are very important. If the counsellor feels uncomfortable it may be very hard for this not to be conveyed to the client. On the other hand, if the counsellor has not been given such strong guidelines about the necessary furniture and is prepared to be flexible, the kind of chairs may well not make all that much difference. Patients in a surgery are probably used to sitting on a hard chair while talking to their GP and thus their expectations about comfort may be a very minor consideration. They have come to see the counsellor to offload their problems and to gain some insight on where they go from here. The counsellor's manner and how well he understands them and accepts them will be far more important than the physical setting.

How chairs are placed is also of some importance. Many GPs nowadays do not sit directly behind their desks with the patient sitting opposite. They may themselves sit behind the desk in order to take notes, but it is likely that the patient's chair is to the side of the desk in a non-confrontational position. For counselling, what is described as the ten-to-two position is often favoured, the two chairs being placed at an angle of about sixty degrees to each other rather than directly facing, for this latter position, even if there is no desk or table in between can be rather threatening. The distance between the chairs is also to be considered. Four or five feet apart is probably about right. If they are closer, that could be too threatening for some clients. If they are too far apart, relating in a meaningful way can be difficult.

Lighting and equipment

Light is also important. If one is counselling someone during the hour when daylight is going to decline, it is better to switch on the light before the session rather than to rise from one's chair to do this during the session. Such an interruption can be distracting. Sometimes when I have forgotten to put the light on before the session, I have allowed the interview to conclude in near darkness rather than interrupt and thus distract from the flow of our meeting.

During daylight hours it is sensible to avoid, if possible, either counsellor or client sitting directly facing the window. To do so means one of the two cannot see the other's face clearly and looking into the light can be uncomfortable.

Some may think that a room such as a doctors' surgery with a good deal of medical equipment in it will interfere with the counselling process. My feeling here is that it certainly can if the counsellor or client believes it will. Both at the college where I worked as part of the counselling team, where the counselling of students took place in the medical centre, and in the GPs' surgery where I have worked for the past eight years, my colleagues and I have often had to see clients in rooms where there has been a medical couch and other equipment. I have no personal evidence that the counselling has been less effective in such settings, nor have those counsellors I have consulted who work in other surgeries. Occasionally I have heard a colleague say that a client has been put off by the medical atmosphere of the setting. For me it is the relationship between counsellor and client that is important, and my belief is that this can be established whatever the physical setup with regard to chairs and other equipment.

The same room each week?

Is it important for the client to see the counsellor in the same room each week? Ideally, this is desirable, since having to change rooms week after week can be distracting, and any unnecessary distraction should be avoided when client and counsellor are looking at emotive and painful issues. However, in a surgery setting it is not always possible to avoid some room changes some of the time and I have personally no clear evidence that clients have been inconvenienced when we have had to meet in a different room from the one we normally have used. Such adaptability is part of everyday experience outside of counselling.

PAYMENT FOR COUNSELLING AND CLIENT MOTIVATION

This is an issue which will not arise where a counsellor is working as a member of the surgery team and all her cases come via the GPs. However, it could arise where, as in the case of our own agency, clients are being seen in a surgery in which the agency is located, rather than being attached. In this particular agency we tell clients that we have expenses and that contributions are welcome. There is no pressure on them to contribute – a number do and others do not.

However, there are those who argue that paying is part of the therapeutic process, that whether it is 50p an hour for those on social security or £30 an hour from someone earning a good salary, the actual commitment to pay as well as to give time is helpful to the client and the work. The difficulty about this argument is that normally when people pay for treatment, for instance for private medical treatment, they are paying for more time, more privacy and for earlier treatment than they might have got as a non-urgent case under the NHS. It is certainly the time and the earlier attention that I have valued on the two occasions in the last twenty years when I have sought such medical help, very well served as I have been on many occasions by the NHS. In counselling, while clients may have to wait for their first appointment because of the increasing demands for the service of a counsellor, once they can be seen they are usually given weekly appointments. Further, having been given an appointment for a particular time, they are seen at that time. What they value is being given time, reliable service and confidentiality. This is what is given in counselling whether they are asked to pay or not.

The motivation of clients is also important in this connection. Clients who are well motivated to change therapeutically are more likely to change. It is also likely to be true that those who are more motivated to change will be more willing to pay for counselling. Thus, when therapists hold the view that payment is part of the therapeutic process, they may well be thinking of those clients who have been willing to pay them. They will probably not have met those unwilling to pay, for whatever reason! But it is not the paying that is primarily responsible for the successful therapy, but the positive motivation of the client, which is more likely to be found in those willing to pay. There is thus no necessary causal connection between payment and the successful outcome of therapy. To consider, again, patients seen under the NHS – a number of these are financially in a position where they could pay had they to do so. But they are not required to pay personally (except through their taxes) and they do not seek private medical treatment. The successful outcome of their treatment could well be accounted for by their positive attitude towards getting better and, where necessary, their willingness to change. Money is a secondary issue and need not be considered a serious part of the 'therapeutic relationship'.

TIME-LIMITED COUNSELLING

The tradition in counselling has been for each interview to last about fifty minutes. While traditions should from time to time be looked at critically, the best grounds for changing this one should be what is best for the client. If a counsellor in discussion with a client feels that a fifty-minute session is unnecessarily long, then it is appropriate to shorten it. However, another reason for shortening sessions may be expediency. Those who are paying for counselling in the surgery, the GPs or whoever else, may require the counsellor to see patients for shorter periods. Some counsellors may resist this and convince the paymasters of the need for the fifty-minute session. Others may at least try shorter sessions. One who did so was Ros Staveley who worked for some nine years in a practice of seven GPs. She writes: 'I was expected to see patients in half-hour slots rather than the recommended hour.' This shorter period forced her to rethink and re-evaluate her techniques and become 'a more directive counsellor (not necessarily a bad thing)' (Staveley 1991: 13).

This greater directiveness meant that in the first session she used a simple questionnaire to obtain information about dependants, marital and occupational status, what difficulties had led the client to see the GP, what the client perceived as 'the problem' and what changes the client would like to see for him or herself or in their life. In less directive counselling such information is almost certainly going to emerge in the course of the interviews. Where time is limited, it can be obtained more quickly by the method Staveley used.

Subsequently, while encouraging the client to 'tell the story' within a Rogerian framework, Staveley used various techniques drawn, for example, from Gestalt therapy and Transactional Analysis, which could involve 'empty-chair work' and role-play which would help clients to experience their feelings more clearly and to clarify their aims. Such techniques can, of course, only be used by counsellors who have confidence in them and feel at ease in using them. They also require clients to be creative, imaginative and quite adventurous. Some clients find this difficult and may need many sessions before they can free themselves from inhibitions and thus be ready to learn experientially.

Being paid by the practice, Staveley had to accommodate herself to the way of working requested by the doctors. She accepted that and makes no suggestion that her counselling of clients for their shorter period (couples were seen for an hour rather than half-an-hour) disadvantaged them. She also tells clients that she usually sees people for six times altogether, and concludes her article: 'I would even go so far as to say the six-session boundary has a cathartic effect in enabling the patient to make changes for him/herself.' Peter Thomas is another counsellor who makes contracts for six sessions and then reviews with the patient, though making his final boundary twenty sessions, after which they would have to see either himself or another counsellor privately. His case study of Anne (1991: 143–5) demonstrates the need for more than six sessions. Having initially talked with Thomas about relationships with men and with her parents, Anne began to explore her need to be in control and to see whether her depression was connected with difficulty in expressing anger and thus losing control. The issues of how Anne controlled men and how this would work out with her male counsellor also had to be explored. Work at that depth does often take considerable time, and in fact the counselling lasted for nearly forty sessions, the last eighteen of which were in private practice. Thomas' account of the course of therapy demonstrates that often many more than six sessions are needed, and sometimes many more than twenty.

House also reports that because of pressures in his surgery, after consultation with the GPs, it was jointly decided to contract with patients for up to six sessions, after which he would help them find counselling elsewhere. He, like Staveley, is having to accommodate his work to take account of the wishes of those who finance the service, but more recently he has been able to negotiate an extension to eight and then ten sessions rather than six. He estimates that about half the clients he sees are helped by eight sessions or fewer, but that at least 15–20 per cent definitely need more.

Other counsellors have found that when they started counselling, their GPs wanted them to limit the number of sessions per client to six. However, they have now convinced their doctors that such limiting is not in the best interests of clients and the doctors have agreed.

Garth, whose surgery is in an area where most of the houses are owned by the council, sees between seven and nine clients per week and originally found that most came for no more than six sessions; thus he had no waiting list. A number came expecting a 'verbal prescription' from him in place of or as well as the GP's prescription for medication. There will always be those clients who wish for a fairly quick solution to their problems. However, recently he has found an increasing number of clients who realise counselling cannot provide a

43

'quick fix' and who are prepared to continue counselling for more than eight sessions.

Other counsellors are conscious of their waiting lists and concerned that clients have to wait for an appointment for several weeks. Sheila finds that a number of her clients want to work at the surface level over their problems. They value being able to discuss them but do not want to work at depth. She feels that they do need support over a period of some weeks, but that such clients, after the first few weeks, do not need to come weekly. She therefore sees these clients fortnightly or over a longer period.

Another method to avoid time-limited counselling is for the counsellor to agree to see some clients without payment. This may be much easier for counsellors who previously worked entirely voluntarily than for those who have paid extensively for their training and whose only or main source of income has been their earnings from their work in Counselling Health Promotion Clinics.

Another way to help over the waiting list is to run groups for clients who have had a number of sessions of individual counselling, and who can see the value of discussing their problems in company with their peers. Peter has run a group for some six clients who had had six individual sessions. The group had six meetings, and although they only met for an hour at a time and attendance was somewhat spasmodic, at the end of the time they opted for a second set of group meetings. Peter feels that all but one of the members gained something from the group, a view about their groups which is shared by Fiona and Richard, who have run three groups for ex-clients in the surgery setting described fully in Chapter 5. While groups are not welcomed by all clients and should only be run for those who have had some individual counselling or have some previous acquaintance of therapeutic groups, the sharing that takes place and the realisation that others have similar problems can enable considerable growth in understanding.

There are thus various strategies to cut down the waiting list; they can also be sensible in themselves. There are clients I have seen for whom I have felt it right that they should decide the date of their next appointment, rather than that I should suggest they come each week. These are clients who have expressed their coping strategies and seem to know what they want to do. They value the support of the counselling meetings when they can talk over their plans for the future; in talking they gain extra clarification for themselves. Similarly, even if there are not the pressures of the waiting list, groups can be of great help to some clients, and it is always worthwhile for counsellors to think about setting up a group if they themselves feel comfortable about facilitating one.

However, there are some problems which clients bring where in the long run it may be very unwise to try to limit their time. These are the cases where clients have experienced a serious breakdown in trust and, particularly, where they have been abused sexually by someone they initially trusted. Sexual abuse, especially for a child or adolescent may have been painful physically but there are types of such abuse which may not have involved physical pain. Nevertheless, the psychological pain may turn out to have been immense. Arthur, for example, may not have felt there was anything wrong when the kindly man who gave him presents and in other ways treated him well wanted to play with his sexual organs, but when Arthur realised later in adolescence what had been going on this affected his whole attitude to adults and his ability to trust them. It would have been most unhelpful in a case of this sort to have limited Arthur to six or eight sessions of counselling – once again trust would have been broken, even if it had been made clear at the outset that there would only be six sessions. Indeed, had he known that, it is possible that Arthur would never have mentioned the abuse at all – it took some sessions before he did reveal it to the counsellor. There may be other cases where it seems appropriate to work at a faster rate, by being more challenging and/or using techniques such as Gestalt where the client might be invited to do some 'empty-chair work' with their pain. George recalls a client who was apparently prepared to go along with this, to help with anger, but who in the following sessions reported that the previous week's session had not been at all helpful. He reports:

> Clearly I was taking the client into a very difficult area for her far earlier than she was ready to go. I see this example as a very clear case of my trying to rush the work, to lead the client rather than following her process, and it could very

well have had disastrous consequences for her. My hunch is that had I not been open to her rejecting the usefulness of this exercise, then she almost certainly would not have come back.

This last remark in itself raises an important issue – the need for the counsellor to make clear that he wishes the client to let him know if he ever says anything or does anything, such as using a technique like that of encouraging the client to 'talk to the empty chair', which seems to the client to be wrong or unhelpful. Openness and honesty are crucial in the counselling process.

There are thus problems about time-limited counselling and even when abuse is not suspected, telling a client that there are only six or eight sessions may mean that it is never mentioned because even that number of sessions is insufficient to enable the client fully to trust the counsellor.

The main question that we are considering, time-limited counselling, is one that has concerned researchers into counselling for some time. Irving and Rowland (1984: 26) for example, found that not all counsellors wished to work in a paid capacity and not all were in favour of becoming part of the NHS, because they felt this would subject them to the same constraints (lack of resources, lack of time and too many clients) as other NHS workers. MacLeod (1988: 6) in her study of fourteen General Practice counsellors, reported that some counsellors felt they were in a stronger position to negotiate and say 'no' to inappropriate referrals when they were not paid by the practice. RELATE counsellors, most of whose work is voluntary and unpaid, are not put under pressure to end their cases before they feel it is appropriate. Similarly, in my own agency which is located in rather than attached to a GPs' surgery, and is described in some detail in Chapter 5, there is no time-limited counselling. Nor of course is there when counsellors work privately and are paid by their clients.

So far, the instances where surgeries are requesting time limits seem to be few in number. But paid counselling in surgeries is still in its infancy. As in the statutory services provided by clinical psychologists and social workers, it is possible that in time pressure may be put on counsellors by those who are paying them. They are likely to resist such pressure, and in the interests of their clients they should do so, but if they succeed they will have achieved something that has not so far proved possible in the statutory services.

THE COUNSELLOR'S WORKLOAD

Counsellors who work full-time are recommended to see not more than twenty clients per week (BAC 1993). Other counsellors who work part-time will agree with their GPs what their total workload should be, but whatever this is, there is liable to be pressure in a surgery for the counsellor to see yet another client and quickly, for the following reason.

It is rare that a patient will have to wait for more than two or three days to obtain an appointment to see the GP of his or her choice. That is the way the surgery works, fairly instant access to help. Patients will of course be aware that unless it is an emergency, they will have to wait weeks if not months for a hospital appointment or to see some specialist outside the surgery, such as a counsellor in an outside agency. But when the counsellor is located in the surgery and is part of the setup there, there is a kind of expectation on the patient's part that they will be given that same kind of quick access as they would get to the nurse or doctor. Even if the GP warns the patient that there is a waiting list for counselling of two to three weeks, there will be some patients whom the GP feels are in need of immediate crisis counselling and so he will be apt to say to the counsellor, 'Could you possibly fit in Mrs A/ Mr B?' The counsellor feels she should, although she has not really got a space; she makes one by staying overtime. And then gradually she begins to realise the pressure on herself due to taking on more work than realistically she should; she needs a very understanding partner in her own home and, possibly, instant access to her counselling supervisor.

One way for a counsellor to overcome this problem of the 'emergency' is to leave one appointment in her weekly programme free for any immediate crisis cases. However, in this connection there is another point. The GP may be understandably convinced that he is dealing with a crisis case which should be seen without delay by the counsellor. However, when the counsellor does give an appointment, the patient is quite calm; there no longer is a great crisis. The very process of airing it with the GP has had more results than the latter anticipated, the 'naming and hearing' with the GP having itself brought great relief. The emergency is past when the client is seen by the counsellor and the counsellor finds herself meeting someone who is in less of a state than some of her regular clients. She thus becomes rather sceptical about crisis counselling, while having to make herself remember that there have been cases where she has felt she has been of great help to a client who has sought immediate counselling.

DISCUSSION ISSUES

1 'We only value what we personally pay for in life.' Do you agree?
2 What have GPs to lose by not prescribing?
3 'Too much flexibility means just being weak.' Is this true in your experience?

4

Does Surgery Counselling Work?

Proof that counselling works (or indeed does harm) is as difficult to ascertain as it would be in psychiatry or any similar discipline. I consider the two kinds of research that have been carried out, along with the limitations of each: (1) objective studies, where measurable criteria such as the number of appointments and prescriptions of psychotropic drugs are used; and (2) subjective studies, where the opinions of clients, counsellors and doctors have been taken into account.

CAN IT BE PROVED THAT SURGERY COUNSELLING 'WORKS'?

This of course is the $64,000 question. It is the same question that can be asked about referral to psychiatrists, psychologists and psychotherapists. The fact that all the practitioners in these three professions are overloaded with cases, despite the increase in their numbers since the war, suggests that their services are needed. But how can this be proved? Psychiatrists and some specially qualified social workers do have statutory duties in that they can if essential 'section' patients. A patient who is behaving in such a way that he or she is putting themselves or others in danger can be hospitalised and, obviously, the power to hospitalise against anyone's will has to be limited to those with special training and expertise. But the vast majority of people with emotional and mental problems do not behave in bizarre or 'mad' ways; they are unhappy, depressed, anxious and occasionally suicidal. The services mentioned above are at full stretch helping them, but the question can still be asked, as of counsellors, how can their services be evaluated and shown to be essential and cost-effective?

One way to prove whether any particular form of treatment works is to compare two similar groups, one of which has the treatment, the other of which does not. When the treatment is by a drug, one group would be given the drug and the other would be given a 'placebo', a substance which the patient is led to believe is the drug but which in fact has no curative properties. But, as Rosalind Corney (1992) points out in a useful chapter on this topic: 'No-one has successfully devised a suitable placebo for therapy.' Thus 'control groups' are those who are put on a waiting list. How many of these feel their problem has been resolved simply due to the passage of time? In our own agency, of some 212 clients who applied for an appointment in ten months in 1992, 166 accepted one when contacted, 25 said they were being helped elsewhere and 21 indicated that the problem had resolved sufficiently for them not to accept. Waiting time before being given an appointment usually varied between three weeks to ten weeks, depending on how easy it was for the client to accept an appointment when one of the team became free. Thus the number who felt the problem had resolved of its own accord over time was only about 10 per cent. It is possible that the problem will recur again and we do have examples of clients who contact us again later. It is also possible that some of those who accepted appointments and received counselling might have reported that their problem had lessened and they felt they no longer needed to come, had they had to wait longer for an appointment. Thus, using those on a waiting list as a 'control group' does not really tell us very much about the likelihood of problems disappearing due to the passage of time and factors other than the counselling. It is very likely that a number of physical problems which patients bring to doctors will also resolve over time without treatment. But these, like mental or emotional ones, may recur later.

Another question that can be asked is whether counselling does any harm. Again the same question can be asked of other forms of treatment such as medication or surgery. Sometimes these treatments are unpleasant and the patient can feel worse, even though the effects of drugs has been thoroughly researched before they are put on the market, and operations can only be carried out by those who have been thoroughly trained. Sometimes, recognised forms of treatment have unpleasant side-effects which the patients are told will have to be endured in the interests of long-term if not immediate health: chemotherapy and radiotherapy, for example. And sometimes, as discussed in Chapter 3, the same drug treatment has unpleasant side-effects for some patients and not for others. So, if we are asking whether counselling is a 'safe' form of treatment, we have to agree that at times clients may feel worse. For example, during the course of an interview, a client may become very tearful or very angry and release those tears and express the anger and for some moments during the interview, feel worse. However, the client may report at the end of the interview that he or she feels better. The tears and the anger needed to be expressed and it was painful, but overall the client benefited. Another possibility in this situation is that the client will not feel better even by the end of the interview but will report that the ensuing week did go better. Again it would seem that the immediate result of the interview was painful, but the later result was beneficial. As already indicated elsewhere, the most crucial thing in counselling is the establishment of trust. One of the reasons why clients may feel worse during an interview or after an interview is their worry about what the counsellor will *really* think of them now. Counsellors may explain confidentiality and may win the client's trust in the first few interviews during which lesser worries are brought out and the client feels accepted and understood. But, probably because of past let-downs by other significant people in her life, the client may have fears whether she will still be accepted now she has revealed *that*. And 'that' in one case could be an abortion carried out even years before, in another a rape where there was some guilt attached, in another, an accident which resulted in serious injury or death. I am often reminded of a client with whom I had built up a good counselling relationship and who had brought up many worrying and unpleasant situations in her earlier life, then suddenly stopped coming after she had revealed her *that*. I kept in contact with her and after some weeks she returned for more counselling. She told me that following the interview when she had revealed *that*, she could not face coming. She felt I might reject her. As far as I could see and as far as I was concerned, she had no grounds for believing this, but she did feel it and she needed time away from counselling. I cannot say I ever understood properly why she felt as she did, but I do not think it in any way realistic to think that any of us, however experienced we are, can ever expect to understand fully why our clients react as they do. The pain that a client may feel during or after an interview or series of interviews cannot therefore be used as a measure of counselling success or failure. It is very difficult to know what measure can be used to indicate harm to a patient.

Thus research into whether counselling is a safe procedure for patients would be very difficult to carry out. A counsellor does not administer drugs or any kind of physical treatment. If, as sometimes does happen, clients find that counselling is becoming emotionally too painful for them, they will be likely to withdraw from it, or at least discuss withdrawal with their counsellor. As we have said, counselling at times will be painful, because the recollection of past traumas and the need to tell the counsellor about them is likely to bring pain as well as relief. However, since the amount of such pain that anyone can bear varies from person to person, to use pain as the measure for whether counselling is safe would be very difficult, if not impossible.

Money and time are more easily measurable, and there have been a number of studies, such as those described below, where these have been used as the measures. Such research can be described as objective, because facts such as the number of prescriptions or the number of surgery attendances are being researched. Other forms of research are subjective, because in these opinions are being asked – of doctors, of counsellors and of patients/clients themselves. Both kinds of research are relevant and necessary.

OBJECTIVE STUDIES

In research of this kind, what is being compared is the number of psychotropic drugs prescriptions and the number of attendances to see the GP before coming for counselling, with the number since coming. In such studies a good researcher will be interested not just in the percentage increase or decrease before and after counselling, but whether the results are statistically significant, i.e., whether such a result is likely simply as a result of chance or not.

Some research is easier to carry out in a surgery setting where GPs have recommended particular patients to seek counselling than in an agency such as RELATE where clients come from many different sources.

It is also desirable that such research is carried out among those patients recommended by GPs, because, as is mentioned in Chapter 1, part of the reason for a GP employing a counsellor is so that he can give more time to those patients whose dis-ease is entirely or mainly physical. Thus it is appropriate to use surgery attendance as a measure. Those who fund the NHS are also interested in costs. As well as the saving of GPs' time, money on medication may also be saved. The kind of drugs that have been measured in such research are those termed psychotropic, which can affect mood and feeling, for example anti-depressants and tranquillisers.

An example of such objective research was that carried out by Dr Stefan Waydenfeld, a GP, and his wife Danuta, a Marriage Guidance Counsellor (1980). Their study involved nine practices, nine counsellors and a total of ninety-nine patients who had been referred by a total of thirty-five GPs, mainly for marital, anxiety and relationship problems. They found that surgery attendance decreased by 31 per cent and psychotropic drug prescriptions by 30 per cent during the period of six months following counselling, compared with six months before it started.

In a study of 84 patients over several years, using similar measures, and carried out in the agency described in Chapter 5, comparing for each one the period since starting counselling to the date of the study with a similar period before starting, I found that the total of attendances dropped from 709 to 605, a drop of nearly 15 per cent. Another finding was that forty-four of these patients attended the surgery fewer times since starting counselling to the date of the study compared with before starting. Twenty-four patients attended more times since starting. Of the thirty-seven patients who had any psychotropic drug prescriptions twenty had fewer such prescriptions after starting compared with before, and seventeen had more.

SUBJECTIVE STUDIES

In these, opinions are sought rather than facts. For example, clients can be asked whether they felt that their counselling helped them and in what way and whether they would themselves recommend counselling to people they know. Doctors can be asked whether they feel patients have been helped by it. In one such study, 75 per cent of patients said that counselling had helped and 82 per cent were said by their GPs to have improved after counselling (Meacher 1977). In another, thirty-five out of fifty-four patients who responded to a questionnaire reported 'general improvement' and had reduced their demand for medical treatment (Anderson and Hasler 1979). In a review of these and other studies, Wyld (1981) concluded that 75 per cent of clients can be expected to show some improvement after being counselled by non-medical workers in a GP setting.

In a study which involved analysing questionnaire responses of fifty-one ex-clients, thirty-five of whom (nearly 70 per cent) responded (Breese 1989), I asked about how well they felt the counsellor had understood them, how much they felt they had been helped, whether they felt the help they had received was still apparent and whether they would recommend the service to others. The responses to these questions were as follows:

The counsellor's understanding
The counsellor showed a good understanding. (26)
The counsellor showed a fair understanding. (9)
The counsellor showed insufficient understanding. (0)

The help received
The counselling helped me a great deal. (17)
The counselling helped quite a bit. (9)
The counselling helped me a little. (8)
The counselling helped hardly at all. (1)

Do you feel the help you received at the time is still apparent?
Yes (28)
No (5)

Would you advise a friend or colleague to seek counselling?
Yes (33)
No (2)

Such figures suggest that the majority of clients appreciated the help they got. We do not, of course, know what the other sixteen clients (30 per cent) who did not respond would have said. They might all have not responded because they did not feel they had been helped, but knowing how such questionnaires through the post are generally received, it is more likely that: (1) some intended to reply but forgot or lost the questionnaire; (2) others disliked any sort of questionnaire and put it straight into the waste-paper basket. It is thus unlikely that any questionnaire study will get much more than a 70 per cent response, and it would not be reasonable to assume that all who did not reply felt that they had not been helped.

Doctors' opinions of the success of counselling are clearly important. An improvement in 88 per cent of cases was reported in the study by the Waydenfelds (1980). A reduction in psychotropic drug prescriptions and in the number of referrals to psychiatrists is also an indication of the value of employing a counsellor and this was found in a study of the estimates of thirty-eight GPs in nine surgeries to which Marriage Guidance counsellors had been attached (Corney 1987: 56).

THE LIMITATIONS OF SUCH STUDIES

When opinions and estimates are asked for, there is always the possibility that the respondent will 'want to please'. Ex-clients may recall that their counsellor was a pleasant person with whom they got on well and thus may want to show their counsellor up in a good light, even though they are told the questionnaire is anonymous and that neither they nor their counsellor will be identified. Doctors may have agreed to use the services of a counsellor and may want to feel that they have made the right decision. Further, when they are asked to estimate whether drug prescriptions have been reduced they may be relying on their memories rather than looking carefully at the patients' records.

In objective studies, if counsellors are being paid for their work, it could be argued that even if money is being saved by fewer prescriptions, the payment of the counsellors may equal the saving of money on prescriptions. Armstrong (1991: 8) asked this question in her article, and states: 'Many psychiatrists, for instance, would say that there is no evidence that counselling is any more effective for anxious and depressed people than anti-depressants given in therapeutic doses for any adequate length of time.' However, against this it has been argued in Chapter 3 that such medication can only reduce symptoms. Counselling will look at the origins of the depression and at possible behaviour change and at ways in which a person's self-image can be improved. This points to the need for long-term research, for looking at surgery attendance and drug prescriptions over years rather than over months. Further, it is indeed possible that during the period when a client is being counselled, emotional pain may for a time increase and necessitate more visits to the GP. This is especially likely when the reason for counselling has been a relationship breakdown or a bereavement. Thus when surgery attendance and drug prescriptions are the measures, what is probably needed is tabulation of the amounts before coming, during the period of counselling and for a period after counselling ends.

Counsellors themselves can help over this by being research-minded and seeing the need for scientific evaluation and publication of their work (Woolfe 1990: 533). There is also the need for large-scale studies conducted by independent researchers to confirm or deny the findings of the small-scale studies quoted in this chapter. It has been suggested that 31 per cent of all General Practices have counsellors and of those which do not, four-fifths would like to have a counsellor, were money and space in their practices available (Sibbald *et al.* 1993: 32). There is thus considerable scope for further studies to ascertain clients' and GPs' opinions of the service provided, and to find out whether counselling has achieved more than alleviation of symptoms and, where relevant, led to the kind of changes in lifestyle that will lead to decrease in heart disease, cancer and suicide and thus contribute to achieving the targets set out in the Government's *Health of the Nation.*

DISCUSSION ISSUES

1 Do you think counselling is an art or a science? How does your answer to this affect the kind of research into counselling that you would carry out?

2   What questions should clients and ex-clients be asked in order to find out how helpful counselling has been?

3   'It's only opinions that really matter. Anything that can be "proved" by statistics should be treated with great suspicion.' Do you agree?

5

Off the Record

An agency located in a GPs' surgery

This chapter begins by tracing the growth of the agency between 1984–92. Training and in-service training, the clients and from where they are referred, the pre-counselling information they are given, how they are received in the surgery and how subsequent appointments are made are then discussed. The chapter concludes with consideration of the administration and finances of the agency, Health Promotion Clinics, some typical cases including a client's view, and how the author sees the possible future of counselling in surgeries.

BEGINNING AND GROWTH

The original inspiration to start this agency came in the mid-1970s when one of our present counsellors, Jocelyn Rawlence, and others were increasingly concerned about the use of drugs among young people. They started a drop-in centre for young people in a location other than our present one and probably chose the name Off the Record because of its implication about confidentiality. It was also the name used by at least two Marriage Guidance Councils in the 1970s which as well as their normal work with older people also saw the need for similar help for young people over personal problems. Over the first few years, Off the Record had various locations and gradually extended the help offered to older people and those with problems unrelated to drugs. It became located in its present premises, a GPs' surgery in a residential area about a mile from the city centre, in the early 1980s.

SINCE 1984

Shortly before taking early retirement/redundancy from my job as a college lecturer employed for the initial training of teachers, and, for my last six years, as course tutor for a Diploma course for teachers wishing also to work as counsellors, I was asked if I would take on the organisation of Off the Record. Told that it was located in a GPs' surgery I immediately agreed, knowing about the value of such locations for counselling, as mentioned in Chapter 1. The senior partner of the GPs, Geoffrey Clayton, saw the surgery 'as a place which the doctors were glad to be fully used for healing'. The counselling in 1984 only took place on a Monday evening and the location, as well as being used for regular agreed clients, had also been advertised as a drop-in centre where anyone calling could be seen immediately. However, it transpired that the drop-in facility had been scarcely used in the previous months, so this was soon given up, since it is wasteful of staff time for counsellors to be waiting for clients if no one turns up.

During the last six months of 1984, there was often insufficient work for the three of us who were counselling on a Monday evening and during the whole of that year only 33 clients were seen for a total of 154 interviews which was in all less than in the previous year, when 45 were seen and 247 interviews were given. We advertised the services in a number of locations and by the end of 1985 had taken on three more counsellors to work at our Norwich surgery on Monday evenings and at other times, while Simon Frey, who had been the organiser of the service in Norwich in the early 1980s, had started working as a counsellor in North Norfolk in a health centre. That year we gave 485 interviews and saw 65 cases.

The next six years saw a steady increase in the number of clients seen in our Norwich centre, an increase in the number of counsellors, and development of the North Norfolk service to six surgeries. 1991 saw the expansion of counselling to a number of other Norwich surgeries including six surgeries in which different members of one team worked. The total number of appointments in 1990, 2,137 (1,118 in our one Norwich location and 1,019 in North Norfolk) had increased in 1992 to 4,516 (2,236 and 2,280 respectively) while another 2,070 appointments were given additionally by our four

Norwich-based counsellors who were also working in other Norwich surgeries.

TRAINING AND IN-SERVICE TRAINING

It is very important that counsellors are trained. What is extremely difficult to know is how long initial training needs to be before trainees start the real work of counselling, and which training courses are better than others. Three of our counsellors who worked with us in the mid-1980s and three of our current team have taken or are taking the two-and-a-half-year part-time course run by Person Centred Therapy (Britain) which brings its members together for training for some nine full days and two residential weeks per year. In addition to the work in groups this course provides for all its members to meet with a tutor for an hour each fortnight for discussion of on-going counselling work and for discussion of their own personal development and also includes a substantial amount of reading and written work. This course is one of the very few courses accredited by the British Association for Counselling. Five others have taken the Certificate Courses in Counselling Skills and in Counselling Theory run by the Central School of Counselling and Therapy, validated by the Associated Examining Board, and four have taken the Diploma Course. Seven others in the team have taken the three-year part-time Certificate Course in Counselling and Groupwork run by the University of Cambridge Board of Extra-Mural Studies. Four others have been trained as RELATE counsellors, another's main training was at the Leo Beck College in London, and another has had training and extensive work as a psychiatric social worker. A number of the team have also taken the introductory courses in counselling at Norwich City College and some of them are currently taking additional part-time courses in Gestalt therapy and body-orientated psychotherapy.

I also subscribe to the notion that no counsellor is ever fully trained. As counsellors we have to consider ourselves permanently arriving rather than having arrived. The same of course should be said of members of all professions.

The on-going in-service training of counsellors is normally given in two ways: the opportunity to meet regularly with colleagues for case discussion; and the opportunity for meeting individually with an experienced counsellor who has also been trained as a supervisor. At Off the Record we have our group meeting twice a month for one-and-a-half hours at lunchtime, or, for those who cannot attend then, on six Saturday mornings a year, and every counsellor has the chance to meet with a supervisor once a month for an hour. Most members of the team take advantage of both these facilities, others are either only able to manage the group or only the individual supervision.

All training courses should do their utmost to ensure that trainees have experience of actual counselling and, well before the end of the course, are counselling 'real' clients under supervision. Counselling has to be learnt primarily by doing; initially by trainees counselling each other and experiencing how they come over by hearing their own audiotapes or seeing videotapes of their actual practice counselling with each other. Such can be very illuminating, especially when discussed in the presence of one's peers and tutors, if at times painful! Counselling training, like being counselled, is no easy option.

THE CLIENTS WE SEE

Of the 258 cases seen at our main surgery in Norwich in 1992, 82 at least brought as their main problem relationships, either an on-going problem with a current partner or with relatives, or with the unhappiness caused by a broken relationship and/or the loneliness that results from not having a relationship, and thirty-four brought as their main problem depression; problems of low self-esteem, panic attacks, anxiety, worry over violence and/or sexual abuse as a child and the problems brought about by difficulties at work and by physical illness each brought five or more clients. Ninety-five clients came as a result of a suggestion from their GP. Forty-two came on the advice of a friend or relative, including ex-clients. Others during 1992 or earlier years came via the CAB, the Norwich Advice Centre, a TV programme, the Well Woman Clinic, RELATE, the Samaritans, two of the other Norwich counselling agencies whose waiting lists were full, a personnel officer at work, MIND, the Conciliation Service, the Student Counselling Service, a social worker, a clinical psychologist, the Occupational Health Centre based at the Norfolk and Norwich

Hospital, Cruse, Victim Support, the Women's Refuge, and the Hamlet Centre and All Saints Centre, two centres in Norwich which help handicapped/disadvantaged people.

Almost all these clients are self-referred in that while counselling may have been recommended to them by one of the above people or agencies, they have had to initiate the process by phoning or writing for an appointment. Very occasionally I have been rung by an agency and have, for some good reason, contacted the client rather than insist the client contacts me.

Some 70 per cent of our clients are women and 30 per cent men. Statistics show that many more women come for counselling than men. Sometimes it is said that women show their emotions more than men do, and it certainly seems that they are readier than men to admit to feeling anxious, depressed and miserable. They may also on the whole be readier to talk about emotions and personal matters than men are and to share with friends or relatives thoughts about personal matters. Showing a stiff upper lip may well be something that some parents require of daughters as much as sons, but perhaps it is on the whole more permissible for small girls to cry and show their emotions than it is for small boys. Counselling involves readiness to talk especially about feelings and perhaps that is the main reason why women are more prepared to come than are men.

THE INFORMATION GIVEN TO POTENTIAL CLIENTS

Figure 1 shows the information slip given by doctors to those patients they recommend to seek counselling, copies of which are also sent to all agencies such as the CAB where people enquire about counselling or which recommend it.

RECEIVING THE CLIENTS AND THE MAKING OF SUBSEQUENT APPOINTMENTS

There will be times when there is a receptionist on duty and the surgery front door will be open. There are other times when the door is locked, the client has to ring for it to be opened, and there is no receptionist. I know of agencies where it is a rule that there must be a receptionist on duty as well

**OFF THE RECORD, NORWICH
COUNSELLING SERVICE
1 Trinity Street,
(Off Unthank Road)
Norwich NR2 2BQ**

Appointments:

These are given Monday to Friday, daytime and evenings. Currently, there is a waiting list, but once clients can be given an appointment they are usually seen weekly.

Fifty minutes is allowed for each appointment.

To get an appointment you can:

either 'phone the organiser on Attleborough (97 from Norwich) 850781. A good time to 'phone is 8.30–9.15 any morning, but you are welcome to try at any other time.

or (if you are a patient at the Trinity St. Surgery) leave a note of your 'phone number or address with the Receptionist. This will be given to the organiser who will 'phone you or write to you and arrange an appointment.

The Service:

Off the Record is a voluntary organisation offering counselling to anyone who wants to talk about personal difficulties, problems over relationships or other issues of concern. The service is confidential and people are seen individually or as a couple if they wish. There is also group counselling for those who would welcome this, normally after they have had individual counselling.

The Aims of Counselling:

Counsellors help people towards a better understanding of their situation and discuss ways in which difficulties can be resolved. Counsellors do not tell people what to do or take responsibility for the actions of others.

Contributions:

Off The Record Counsellors have all had training and work to a professional standard. Much of our work is done without pay, but the service has expenses and clients are asked to give as generously as they can.

Figure 1 Information slip given by doctors to those patients they recommend to seek counselling.

as the counsellor before counselling is allowed. I can understand this rule and in such an agency I would abide by it. However where we work, we have not yet seen the need to employ a special receptionist during the hours when the surgery is closed. We have yet to have clear evidence that such is essential. We do try to ensure that there are at least two counsellors working during those hours when there is no receptionist on duty, though we do not always achieve this.

During the hours when surgery is on, a client will be asked to report to the receptionist and say they have a counselling appointment with the particular counsellor whose name they have been given. The counsellor, rather as the GPs do, will go into the waiting area and call the name of the client. There is no particular reason for other patients to know whether the person who has been called is there for a medical interview or a counselling interview. Following the first interview, the normal practice is for the counsellor, who now knows what the client looks like, to enter the waiting area and quietly make some signal to the client rather than call out the name. There is no evidence of any difficulty or embarrassment for clients over this procedure. On the other hand I do know of an agency where trouble is taken to ensure that clients have no contact with each other, for fear of recognition or possible embarrassment. Perhaps this last is more likely in a specialist counselling agency where all who come are coming for the same purpose than in a surgery where some are coming to see a doctor, others are coming to see the practice nurse and yet others are coming for a counselling appointment.

As regards the making of the appointments, the task of arranging the initial appointment is done usually on the phone by myself from my home. I arrange appointments for over two hundred clients a year currently, a considerable increase on the number I arranged when I first took over the agency. It is only rarely that a client fails to turn up for a first appointment. Subsequent appointments are made by the counsellor with the client and are entered in the appointments book. The information given to the counsellor is the client's name, address and phone number, how the client came to know of the agency and any other details the client has given to me. On the few occasions I have received a referral letter from a doctor or a specialist I have also passed this to the counsellor.

Even if clients have been recommended by a doctor, it is they who have made the appointment. Thus they are all self-referred. I do not recommend that other members of the counselling team give their phone numbers to clients, though some do this. Very occasionally a counsellor who has done so has regretted it because the client has taken advantage and has phoned them too often and at very inconvenient times.

ADMINISTRATION OF THE WORK OF THE AGENCY

My predecessors as organisers had publicised their home phone numbers and were contacted at home by potential clients. This was a similar procedure to the one I recall in North Hertfordshire when I first became a Marriage Guidance counsellor in the 1960s, the appointments secretary being someone who worked from her home. I was aware that Marriage Guidance (now RELATE) Centres had long since changed that procedure and had appointments secretaries working during office hours at the Centre's headquarters. However, I was willing to adopt the existing Off the Record system when I took over in 1984 and receive calls from would-be clients at home. While the work has increased over the years to the point where I am likely to have on average five incoming phone calls each weekday and am likely to make five, adding up to three hours on the phone a week, and also have to write the occasional letter to clients who are not on the phone or who never seem to be in when phoned (probably about two dozen a year), I do not yet find the appointments secretary side of the work too cumbersome. We have at home an answerphone to help us, my wife takes calls and sometimes has to act on them when I am out, and when we are away there is provision for one of my colleagues in the agency to make appointments and receive calls. I have to say that I can recall no instances of abuse of the phone during the past eight years. Occasionally I have had a call late at night or during Sunday lunch – that is all. Ironically there was more abuse in the years when I first worked as a Marriage Guidance counsellor and did not publicise my phone number! I recall during six years there three occasions when clients found my address in the phone book and rang me at inconvenient times and were in other respects a small nuisance.

Other administration of the service consists of collecting statistics from colleagues at the end of each year to write the Annual Report which is circulated to doctors and others who refer clients, writing progress reports and requests for information of one kind or other to members of the team, responding to the occasional request from the local media and keeping details of which clients are currently being seen by each counsellor and of those on the waiting list who will be needing appointments – all this via a very simple card index system. Administration could be more thorough – I could keep a record of every incoming and outgoing phone call, I could keep strictly to office hours, I could always have letters etc. professionally typed – I could work from an office located in the Centre.... I choose to work from home in a study and I have a very understanding and considerate wife who is always prepared to help this growing service to the community. Working as I do, I can phone clients who work during the day in the evenings when they are more likely to be at home.

FINANCES

The Annual Report for 1986 stated: 'Our very modest expenses for travel, subscription to the British Association for Counselling, fees, stationery, postage and telephone amounted for the year to £167 and were met mainly from donations given by members of the team for work done outside the Agency.' At that time we were not allowed even to suggest to our clients that they give us donations. The doctors in whose surgery we worked insisted on that as a condition for our working there. However, in the last two years, since it has become possible for counsellors in other surgeries to receive remuneration for Health Promotion Clinics mentioned below, that rule has been relaxed. Thus in 1989 we were able to report that we were receiving donations from a number of clients and were able to consider paying a mileage allowance to those counsellors who had to travel into Norwich. In 1990, initially that mileage allowance was 10p a mile but by 1991 that had increased to 20p, its present amount. Discussion with the Family Health Services Authority in Norwich (then known as the Family Practitioner Committee) in 1990 led to them giving a grant of £2,000 for that year to help us with travel, printing, photocopying and postage expenses, subscriptions to BAC and for certain journals, payment to our clinical psychologist consultant who comes to our lunchtime case discussion group six times a year, and for grants to our counsellors for extra training. Our income for that year amounted to £3,367.50 and expenditure to £3,537.63. Up to and including that year most of the individual supervision had been done by myself and I had received no payment for it. In 1991, with the growth of the work and its extension into other surgeries, payment for supervision whether by myself or by outside supervisors was regularised. Income rose to £7,836.14, client contributions amounting to £2,902.35, the grant from the FHSA to £2,000, a donation to £200, while £2,400 came from the Health Promotion Counselling Clinics which were run for those patients who came to us from our doctors' own particular surgeries and where at least two patients could be seen by the same counsellor in the same period of time. Expenditure that year came to £8,081.15, consisting of £3,415.42 for travel expenses, £1,351.66 for supervision, £744 as grants to counsellors for extra training courses and £1,854 to those counsellors who gave more than a hundred interviews. Consultant's fee, insurance, subscriptions, printing, postage, phone bills, photocopying, and certain necessary purchases made up the rest of the expenditure.

HEALTH PROMOTION CLINICS

In 1990 the NHS started very openly to encourage GPs to think in terms of promoting good health rather than only giving treatment after illness had started. The idea that 'prevention is better than cure' makes sound sense. Through the Family Health Services Authority which supervises primary health care, GPs were encouraged to put on special clinics, run by themselves or other staff, for conditions like hypertension, smoking cessation, alcohol awareness, stress management, asthma, coronary heart disease risk reduction screening and counselling services. In such clinics patients would come for regular check-ups and treatment where necessary outside the usual surgery hours. Payment would be given for these clinics, provided a specified number of patients were seen and the clinic lasted for a specified period. The Norwich FHSA agreed that counselling could be one of the Health Promotion

Clinics that could be run in a surgery under the supervision of the GPs, and in 1991 an increasing number of GPs began to employ counsellors to run counselling clinics. The criteria were that at least two clients must be seen currently by the same counsellor who should either have accreditation from the British Association for Counselling or have had appropriate training of at least 450 hours, should receive regular on-going supervision, work to a written code of ethics and preserve client confidentiality.

So popular and thus expensive did Health Promotion Clinics become that by the start of 1992 FHSAs were having to have second thoughts about them and now (July 1993) such clinics for counselling have ended.

The emphasis in health promotion from now on is to be on reaching the Government targets, as set out in the leaflet *The Health of the Nation*, i.e., to reduce coronary heart disease, strokes, cancers, smoking, suicide and accidents particularly. It may not be easy to prove conclusively that counselling can help substantially to achieve these targets, though I am sure all counsellors can produce evidence from clients that counselling has reduced the stress that is clearly associated with heart disease and the other conditions and that it has also helped to reduce the likelihood of accidents and suicide attempts. Currently counselling can be funded under the scheme whereby GPs can claim 70 per cent reimbursement for ancillary workers. However, even this may not be possible after March 1994. While very many GPs value the work of counsellors in their surgeries, not all of them are prepared to put a greater value on counselling than on their other necessary ancillary services.

There is also the question of how the payment of counsellors should compare with that of other surgery staff. Those of our team who were also working in other surgeries were able in 1992 to negotiate fees which range between £12 per hour and £18, the amount depending on the particular contract each had. If the necessary funding can eventually become available, it is likely that more surgeries will be willing to pay for the services of a counsellor, as the research carried out by Sibbald *et al.*, mentioned in Chapter 4, suggests. In a report by the health correspondent of the Norwich-published newspaper, the *Eastern Daily Press* (7 February 1992), the Chairman of the

Norfolk Local Medical Committee, Dr Brian Elvy, is quoted as saying that most doctors were now well aware of the value of counselling services and he advised patients to turn to them whenever necessary. He went on to say 'Doctors are given much better training on the counselling aspect of the job, but what we simply do not have is the time', the point made also by our own GP contributors to this book in earlier chapters.

So, whether the necessary funding will eventually become available is very much in the balance. Sue Vaughan, the senior partner at the surgery where Off the Record is located sums up the situation as follows:

> The future relationship between GPs and counsellors from the financial point of view is unclear. Nineteen ninety-three has seen the end of the present system of payments to GPs for running Health Promotion Clinics which has allowed a rapid expansion of counselling services in Norfolk (although not in all parts of the country. The rules have been interpreted in an imaginative way by the Norfolk Family Health Services Authority.) Staff budgets for GPs will probably not stretch to allow direct employment of counsellors if that means not being able to employ as many receptionists or other staff more directly involved in the day-to-day work of the practice. Money for GP services is set to dwindle as budgets are pared down. How many counsellors can afford to go back to providing their services free? And indeed why should they, given the clear need for their services? A case needs to be made for the purchase of counselling services as part of the basic spectrum of health services needed by the community. How much counselling do the people of Norfolk need and how much should be spent on counselling compared with all other types of health care? Difficult questions to answer or even to know who should do the answering!

SOME TYPICAL CASES

Angela, a client with what were initially just physical problems was recommended by her GP to seek counselling, because she admitted also to being depressed. The counsellor could well understand how someone with these particular physical problems would be depressed because they were extremely frustrating for the client – she was unable to do any of the things that she wanted to do. She had a supportive and understanding partner, but she also felt it was helpful to come for counselling because she did not want to overburden her partner with her problems. She found it helpful to share these with the counsellor, even thought there was little likelihood of a solution being found, at least in the near future.

Jane was recommended for counselling because of her anxiety, panic attacks and worries that she might be going mad. She had also asked to see a psychiatrist and had been given an appointment for some ten weeks hence, about eight weeks after her counselling started. She needed a listener who took her seriously, unlike her mother, who had been inclined to dismiss her problem and suggest ways of coping with it that did not appeal to her. In accepting her and in understanding how she felt, the counsellor was assuring her at least of her sanity, that she was not mad to feel the way she did. She, like the previous client mentioned, felt supported and understood, while she and the counsellor looked at various alternatives for action to ease the emotional pain she was experiencing.

Walter had had a stroke, which among other things prevented him from driving, an activity he much enjoyed. He had some very supportive friends who gave him a great deal of help which he much appreciated, but he needed to talk over his feelings about not being able to drive, as well as the hopes he had of being assessed at a special centre in order to see whether he would be able to drive a suitably adapted car. He found talking to the counsellor for about six sessions a considerable help and both he and the latter rejoiced when he had been successfully assessed and was able to look forward to driving again. The opportunity to share his thoughts, feelings and wishes may well have given him the confidence he needed when going for the assessment.

Philip and Mary came with Ian, their 15-year-old son. He had been truanting from school, had been stealing from them and was generally disaffected. He had been a very promising athlete who it seemed might be capable of the highest honours in his chosen sport. His parents had spent both time and money in helping him and for several years he had been very happy with this sport. But recently he had lost interest and turned to another sport which he was now far more keen to pursue. The reason for his change in behaviour at home and school seemed to be linked with the fact that he wanted his parents to accept his change of heart rather than continue to hanker after his being successful in the previous sport. It sounded to the counsellor that they were wanting him to lead his life their way because of the glory it might bring them as the parents of a very successful athlete. Some three sessions, in which Ian was able to express his feelings and and be accepted, seemed to help the relationship between him and his parents a great deal, and they found they could accept his change of interest and not hold the time and money they had previously spent on his behalf against him.

Joan, in her twenties, having left school without very much in the way of exam successes, was thinking of higher education and was taking a quite taxing college course with a view to this. She had a need to talk through her current relationship with her parents and friends, particularly her need to be firmer with a friend who tended to take advantage of her, and also her college work situation and her worries about the exams she was to take. As with Walter, both she and the counsellor shared some joy when she was able to report she had been successful and could now look to the future with more confidence.

Annabel was older than Joan and successful both in her work and as a wife and mother, yet she felt there was a black cloud around her which was making her depressed. As she began talking with the counsellor, she began to feel it was related very much to her own family situation some twenty years before when she felt she had not been fairly treated by her father, especially when compared with her sisters and brother. The reasons for this were fully discussed and she had the choice to try to talk to her parents and explain her feelings to them. In the event, she chose not to because she did not want to hurt them and because she felt they still would not really understand. However, the eight or so sessions of counselling enabled the black cloud to lift somewhat and she felt less depressed about the situation.

Alice came because she felt she had been terribly let down by the man with whom she had lived for some eight years and who had now formed a relationship with a younger woman. He was actually several thousand miles away when she came, but she still had a great need to phone him and appeal to him. She was very tearful and desperate – several times during the weeks she came for counselling, she phoned the Samaritans and obtained much-needed and helpful support from them. Over the weeks of counselling she began to express her anger as well as her tears and the phone calls to her ex-partner decreased. Finally she was able to obtain a job and began to look forward to a life without the man in an entirely new area. For her, and for so many other clients in similar situations who feel they have been badly let down and lost someone very important to them, this was worse than a bereavement. When someone dies, they are, as it were, inaccessible, and they have not rejected one in preference to another human being. The feelings of the one abandoned of disappointment, frustration, rejection and misery are very considerable. Time usually heals the wound to some extent, and the presence of a counsellor during the weeks of misery is a kind of hand-holding operation in which the feelings can be outpoured. Getting angry and expressing that anger fully seems a necessary part of the process until time eventually allows for healing and, maybe even eventually, forgiveness.

These seven cases are perhaps typical of those one may meet within surgery counselling. In two of them there was physical disability as well as the feelings of frustration that can accompany this. In the others the predominant feelings were those of being misunderstood and let down by other significant people. By being there, by being reliable, and above all by being human, the counsellor helped them at a crucial time when they were needing to share and needed to be fully understood.

A CLIENT'S VIEW OF THE SERVICE

Following the publication of our Annual Report for 1991, I was contacted by the *Eastern Daily Press*, whose health correspondent was particularly keen to publicise the help that was available in agencies such as ours for people who were depressed, this in the context of the press reports that the Royal College of Psychiatrists and the Royal College of General Practitioners have launched a five-year campaign, Defeat Depression. I was asked if I could find a client who had recently received counselling whom the health correspondent could contact. The first ex-client I phoned said she would rather not be contacted. The second one, Karen, agreed and what she had to say was reported in the newspaper on 7 February 1992 as follows:

I had been through a terrible experience and when it really hit me what had happened, I was completely confused and just didn't know what to do. It is impossible to describe the feeling. It took over everything. The counselling helped me to step back a few paces and look at what was going on without being so involved. It gave me back my self-confidence. Off the Record is a wonderful organisation. It is extremely important that they are there, especially for the many people who have no family network to turn to for help when they really need it.

She had been advised to seek counselling by her GP and said that it took a year of counselling before she felt she had 'turned the corner'. She was seen weekly to start with and then at less frequent intervals, for a total of nineteen interviews altogether.

THE GP PERSPECTIVE

Sue Vaughan, senior partner at the surgery, writes:

It is difficult to recall a time when Off the Record counsellors were not using our rooms when not needed for surgeries. So referral to a counsellor has been fairly straightforward for a long time and we have certainly offered this option to many of our patients. Who do we select for referral and what can we say about the outcome?

Estimates of the proportion of patients consulting GPs whose main problem, whatever the presenting symptoms, is an underlying psychological difficulty range up to 30 per cent. How the GP tackles the consultation will reflect his own need to be sure significant organic problems have been excluded. Exploration of areas in the patient's life that could be the source of psychological distress can be revealing for both patient and doctor but entails the risk that more may be revealed than can be decently dealt with in a five to ten minute slot. How many clues the doctor follows up will depend on how tightly he is constrained by the need to be reasonably on time. Always being thirty minutes late with appointments is frowned upon by other patients who have read the Patient's Charter. Nevertheless, the moment that a patient reveals an area of pain has a quality that is difficult to recapture when they return for a longer appointment at a more convenient time. So many of us can't resist staying with the moment and doing our own form of counselling there and then.

Sadly, for the majority of our patients, there just is not the time for more than a brief assessment of the psychological factors behind their symptoms and the GP uses this assessment to decide on the likely value of more extensive work with someone else. The counselling service is the first choice for the majority whose lives are in a muddle with relationship problems, past or present, or who need help to take stock, our so-called neurotics. The suggestion that counselling could be helpful is much more readily accepted these days and indeed, more and more patients skip the preliminary physical presentation and come to ask for referral to a counsellor. (There are no posters advertising the service around our waiting room, but information slips are readily available.)

For patients with evidence of significant depression or anxiety, a blend of drug treatment with counselling is often the course chosen by our doctors and we continue monitoring the response to drugs in tandem with attendance at counselling sessions.

It would be interesting to analyse whom we refer where and why we choose a counselling instead of a psychiatric or psychological service and vice versa. One problem in carrying out such a study would be the informal nature of our referrals to counsellors. It takes the form of giving the patient the details of how to contact Off the Record and only rarely do we write any form of referral letter. There is also no feedback from the counsellor unless there is concern over deteriorating mental health. So we don't know how often our suggestion that counselling would help is acted on by the patient or what the outcome is in the majority of cases. This is in contrast to referrals to psychiatrists where there are detailed letters back and forth. This difference underlies the choice of counselling for many patients for whom the recording of so much information about their private lives in a less than totally confidential way feels inappropriately intrusive.

In assessing how much patients have benefited from counselling, we are up against the problem of the long time-span of change and finding out what has been of most help in allowing change to occur. I think we have to trust the patients and undoubtedly many report that it was very helpful to them to see a counsellor. We also have patients who say it was no help. The reasons for this are no doubt many and varied.

THE FUTURE

Counselling is becoming more of a paid profession, although at present there are still national agencies like RELATE and the Catholic Marriage Advisory Council, and local agencies such as, in Norwich, the St Barnabas Centre for Counselling and Off the Record, where the majority of the work is done voluntarily, though to a professional standard. As I have already indicated elsewhere, one advantage of working voluntarily is that the pace of work can be one's own. Counsellors can give the time to each of their clients that they and the client feel is appropriate, initially weekly appointments of fifty minutes in most instances. For this reason they may be the envy not only of doctors, who may well be seeing ten patients in an hour rather than one, but also of social workers, clinical psychologists and others in the helping professions who, because they are paid, must, inevitably, have their case-loads to some extent determined by those who pay them. Professionals who work either wholly or partly privately can also, of course, determine their case-loads. While it is very understandable that many counsellors should wish to be paid for their work, either because pay is a necessity for them to live or because pay is a mark of recognition that the work is worthwhile, they may well have to expect pressure, as has happened in social and psychological work, to see clients less frequently and as mentioned in Chapter 3, for shorter times. If they can resist such pressure, they will have succeeded where other professions have not.

People sometimes ask me why there has been this considerable growth in counselling in surgeries in recent years and what people did before there was so much counselling. I believe the increase in demand is partly due to the recession, in which there are not jobs for all who wish for them, jobs not only relieving financial problems but also giving people a sense of purpose. But more than this, the fact that so many of the problems brought are because of unhappiness over relationships suggests to me that a greater problem than the recession is the greater choice people have over their behaviour. The more choice available, the more complex life becomes. People want to be able to trust one another and be trusted, but trust can be damaged by selfishness: the man who has been let down, often in his early friendships, has difficulty in trusting his present partner, while she resents his lack of trust and arguments start which can lead to violence. The woman who gave herself early in her life to someone whom she felt really loved her and then was let down by him, over time enters into other relationships. Again she is let down and comes to counselling wondering what it is that always results in her becoming involved with what she feels is the wrong sort of man. These sorts of problems are the ones that are constantly coming to counsellors, having led to a loss of confidence and to low self-esteem, a characteristic described by Seamands (1981: 49) as 'Satan's deadliest weapon'. Such a description may sound exaggerated, but counsellors, whether Christian or not, will agree that helping people to combat low self-esteem is quite a task.

As to what people did before: while many clients seem to be looking for their counsellor to be a more understanding parent than they felt their own parents were, it certainly seems from what clients say that the greater incidence of divorce has created more confusion in the minds of children and adolescents about standards of behaviour than there was before, a confusion which is with them in adulthood, when they still need parental support. Furthermore, even for clients whose parents stayed contentedly together, the tendency for the next generation to live farther afield from parents and grandparents means that when support is needed, access to it is harder than it used to be.

The role of the counsellor as understanding, encouraging and non-judgemental parent is one that counsellors working in a secular setting find themselves adopting. If they themselves are non-believers they will not want to bring God into it, and even those who believe in God may feel it is inappropriate to mention biblical teaching. But it is perhaps more than a coincidence that on the day I was concluding this chapter I found myself reading the passage in St Paul's Epistle to the Philippians (2: 3–7) where he speaks of Christ taking the very nature of a servant and of the importance of humility, while the previous day's reading in the first Epistle to the Corinthians, Paul wrote of the need for adaptability (1 Cor.: 19–23). The good counsellor has to be adaptable, caring and servant-like in the sense of being non-authoritarian. Those with emotional problems will, it seems to me, always need people with such an attitude.

DISCUSSION ISSUES

1 Should counsellors be prepared to work voluntarily?
2 Do you think the training of counsellors should be standardised in the same kind of way that the training of teachers, doctors and other professionals is?
3 Given the choice, and being told that both were equally good, would you choose for yourself a counsellor of the same sex or of the opposite sex?
4 To what do you attribute the increase in the need for counselling?

Further Reading

Bennett, P. (1993), *Counselling for Heart Disease*, British Psychological Society: Leicester.

British Association for Counselling (1993), *Counselling in General Practice: A New Guide for Counsellors and GPs*, BAC: Rugby.

Dale, P. (1993), *Counselling Adults who were Abused as Children*, BAC: Rugby.

Dryden, W. and Feltham, C. (1992), *Brief Counselling*, Open University Press: Milton Keynes.

Hammersley, D. (forthcoming 1994), *Counselling People on Prescribed Drugs*, Sage: London.

Mearns, D. and Dryden, W. (1989), *Experience of Counselling in Action*, Sage: London.

Ross, A. (1990), *Helping the Depressed*, Kingsway: Eastbourne.

Sheldon, M. (ed.) (1992), *Counselling in General Practice*, Royal College of General Practitioners Clinical Series: Exeter.

Street, E. (forthcoming 1994), *Counselling for Family Problems*, Sage: London.

Waskett, C. (1993), *Counselling in Eating Distress*, BAC: Rugby.

References

CHAPTER 1

Basharan, H., Einzig, H. and Jenkins, G. C. (1992), 'The Training Needs of Counsellors Working in Primary Medical Care: The Role of Training Organisations', BAC Counselling in Medical Settings *Newsletter* 33, pp. 9–13.

Dickson, D. A. (1989), 'Interpersonal communication in the health professions: a focus on training', *Counselling Psychology Quarterly*, vol. 2(3), pp. 345–66.

Heisler, J. (1979), 'Marriage counsellors in medical settings', *Marriage Guidance*, vol. 18(5), pp. 153–62.

Hudson, G. (1988), 'Counsellors within General Practice: time and need for utilization, credibility and accreditation', BPS Counselling Psychology Section *Review* vol. 3(1), pp. 15–20.

McLeod, J. (1988), *The Work of Counsellors in General Practice*, Royal College of General Practitioners Occasional Paper 37.

Morrell, V. (1992), 'Developing counselling skills', in M. Sheldon (ed.), *Counselling in General Practice*, Royal College of General Practitioners Clinical Series: Exeter, pp. 15–19.

Rowland, N. (1992), 'Counselling and counselling skills', in M. Sheldon (ed.), *Counselling in General Practice*, Royal College of General Practitioners Clinical Series: Exeter, pp. 1–7.

——, Irving, J. and Maynard, A. (1990), 'Can General Practitioners counsel?', *Journal of the Royal College of General Practitioners*, vol. 39, pp. 118–20.

CHAPTER 2

De Groot, M. (1985), *Marriage Guidance Counsellors in the Medical Setting*, Research Report 1, Marriage Guidance Council: Rugby, p. 17.

Garlton, C. (1992), 'A receptionist's perspective', in M. Sheldon (ed.), *Counselling in General Practice*, Royal College of General Practitioners Clinical Series: Exeter, p. 35.

References

Irving, J. (1992), 'The practice counsellor', in M. Sheldon (ed.), *Counselling in General Practice*, Royal College of General Practitioners Clinical Series: Exeter, pp. 26–9.

McLeod, J. (1988), *The Work of Counsellors in General Practice*, Royal College of General Practitioners Occasional Paper 37.

Rowland, N. and Hurd, J. (1991), *Counselling in General Practice, A Guide for Counsellors*, BAC Counselling in Medical Settings Division, p. 6.

CHAPTER 3

British Association for Counselling (1993), *Guidelines for the Employment of Counsellors in General Practice*, BAC: Rugby, p. 21.

Hammersley, D. and Beeley, L. (1992), 'The effect of medication on counselling', *Counselling*, vol. 3(3), pp. 162–4.

Irving, J. and Rowland, N. (1984), 'The future of General Practice counselling', *Counselling*, no. 50, BAC, pp. 23–8.

McLeod, J. (1988), *The Work of Counsellors in General Practice*, Royal College of General Practitioners Occasional Paper 37.

Staveley, R. (1991), 'An evaluation of short-term counselling', BAC Counselling in Medical Settings *Newsletter* 26, pp. 13–17, and personal correspondence 1993.

Thomas, P. (1991), 'A therapeutic journey through the garden of Eden', *Counselling*, vol. 2(4), pp. 143–5.

CHAPTER 4

Armstrong, E. (1991), 'A new miracle worker? A critical look at counselling in General Practice', BAC Counselling in Medical Settings *Newsletter* 29, pp. 7–9.

Anderson, S. and Hasler, J. C. (1979), 'Counselling in General Practice', *Journal of the Royal College of General Practitioners*, vol. 29, pp. 352–6.

Breese, J. H. (1989), 'Obtaining feedback from clients', BPS Counselling Psychology Section *Review*, vol. 4(1), pp. 14–16.

Corney, R. H. (1987), 'Marriage guidance counsellors in General Practice in London', *British Journal of Guidance and Counselling*, vol. 15(1), pp. 50–8.

Meacher, M. (1977), *A Pilot Scheme with General Practitioners*, The Mental Health Foundation.

Sibbald, B., Addington-Hall, J., Brenneman, D. and Freeling, P. (1993), 'Counsellors in English and Welsh General Practices: their nature and distribution', *British Medical Journal*, vol. 306, pp. 29–33.

Waydenfeld, D. and Waydenfeld, S. W. (1980), 'Counselling in General Practice', *Journal of the Royal College of General Practitioners*, vol. 30, pp. 671–7.

References

Woolfe, R. (1990), 'Counselling psychology in Britain: an idea whose time has come', *The Psychologist*, vol. 3(12), pp. 531–5.

Wyld, K. L. (1981), 'Counselling in General Practice: a review', *British Journal of Guidance and Counselling*, vol. 1(2), pp. 129–41.

CHAPTER 5

Seamands, D. A. (1981), *Healing for Damaged Emotions*, Victor Books: Wheaton, Illinois, p. 49.

Index